Enhancing Scientific Reproducibility in Biomedical Research Through Transparent Reporting

PROCEEDINGS OF A WORKSHOP

Theresa Wizemann, Sylvia Ncha, Amanda Wagner Gee, and
Carolyn Shore, *Rapporteurs*

Forum on Drug Discovery, Development, and Translation
Forum on Neuroscience and Nervous System Disorders
National Cancer Policy Forum
Roundtable on Genomics and Precision Health

Board on Health Sciences Policy
Board on Health Care Services

Health and Medicine Division

The National Academies of
SCIENCES · ENGINEERING · MEDICINE

THE NATIONAL ACADEMIES PRESS
Washington, DC
www.nap.edu

THE NATIONAL ACADEMIES PRESS **500 Fifth Street, NW Washington, DC 20001**

This activity was supported by contracts between the National Academy of Sciences and AbbVie Inc.; Amgen Inc. (Contract No. GHCCOPS-CSARF-175837); Association of American Medical Colleges; AstraZeneca; Burroughs Wellcome Fund (Contract No. 1020264); Cell Press; Critical Path Institute; Eli Lilly and Company; FasterCures; Foundation for the National Institutes of Health; Friends of Cancer Research; GlaxoSmithKline (Contract No. 016084); Johnson & Johnson; The Lancet; Merck & Co., Inc. (Contract Nos. CMO-180308-002499 and MRL-CPO-18-2641); National Institutes of Health (Contract No. HHSN263201800029I; Task Order Nos. HHSN26300007 and HHSN26300009): National Cancer Institute, National Center for Advancing Translational Sciences, National Institute of Allergy and Infectious Diseases, National Institute of Mental Health, National Institute of Neurological Disorders and Stroke, Office of Extramural Research, Office of Science Policy; Nature Research; *New England Journal of Medicine*; Sanofi (Contract No. 44723099); Takeda Pharmaceuticals (Contract No. 398929); and U.S. Food and Drug Administration (Grant Nos. 5R13FD005496-04 and 5R13FD005496-05): Center for Drug Evaluation and Research and Office of the Commissioner. Any opinions, findings, conclusions, or recommendations expressed in this publication do not necessarily reflect the views of any organization or agency that provided support for the project.

International Standard Book Number-13: 978-0-309-66349-6
International Standard Book Number-10: 0-309-66349-0
Digital Object Identifier: https://doi.org/10.17226/25627

Additional copies of this publication are available from the National Academies Press, 500 Fifth Street, NW, Keck 360, Washington, DC 20001; (800) 624-6242 or (202) 334-3313; http://www.nap.edu.

Printed in the United States of America

Suggested citation: National Academies of Sciences, Engineering, and Medicine. 2020. *Enhancing scientific reproducibility in biomedical research through transparent reporting: Proceedings of a workshop.* Washington, DC: The National Academies Press. https://doi.org/10.17226/25627.

The National Academies of
SCIENCES · ENGINEERING · MEDICINE

The **National Academy of Sciences** was established in 1863 by an Act of Congress, signed by President Lincoln, as a private, nongovernmental institution to advise the nation on issues related to science and technology. Members are elected by their peers for outstanding contributions to research. Dr. Marcia McNutt is president.

The **National Academy of Engineering** was established in 1964 under the charter of the National Academy of Sciences to bring the practices of engineering to advising the nation. Members are elected by their peers for extraordinary contributions to engineering. Dr. John L. Anderson is president.

The **National Academy of Medicine** (formerly the Institute of Medicine) was established in 1970 under the charter of the National Academy of Sciences to advise the nation on medical and health issues. Members are elected by their peers for distinguished contributions to medicine and health. Dr. Victor J. Dzau is president.

The three Academies work together as the **National Academies of Sciences, Engineering, and Medicine** to provide independent, objective analysis and advice to the nation and conduct other activities to solve complex problems and inform public policy decisions. The National Academies also encourage education and research, recognize outstanding contributions to knowledge, and increase public understanding in matters of science, engineering, and medicine.

Learn more about the National Academies of Sciences, Engineering, and Medicine at **www.nationalacademies.org**.

PLANNING COMMITTEE ON ENHANCING SCIENTIFIC REPRODUCIBILITY IN BIOMEDICAL RESEARCH THROUGH TRANSPARENT REPORTING[1]

HARVEY FINEBERG (*Chair*), Gordon and Betty Moore Foundation
OTIS BRAWLEY, Johns Hopkins University
BARRY COLLER, The Rockefeller University
STUART HOFFMAN, Department of Veterans Affairs
VERONIQUE KIERMER, PLOS
BENEDICT KOLBER, Duquesne University
ALEXA McCRAY, Harvard Medical School
JILL MESIROV, University of California, San Diego School of Medicine
MARTIN MURPHY, CEO Roundtable on Cancer
RICHARD NAKAMURA, Center for Scientific Review, National Institutes of Health (*Retired*)
FRANKLIN SAYRE, Thompson Rivers University
IDA SIM, University of California, San Francisco
VALDA VINSON, *Science*

Health and Medicine Division Staff

CAROLYN SHORE, Director, Forum on Drug Discovery, Development, and Translation
AMANDA WAGNER GEE, Program Officer
SYLVIA NCHA, Associate Program Officer
MELVIN JOPPY, Senior Program Assistant
ANDREW M. POPE, Senior Director, Board on Health Sciences Policy

Consultant

THERESA WIZEMANN, Science Writer

[1] The National Academies of Sciences, Engineering, and Medicine's planning committees are solely responsible for organizing the workshop, identifying topics, and choosing speakers. The responsibility for the published Proceedings of a Workshop rests with the workshop rapporteurs and the institution.

FORUM ON DRUG DISCOVERY, DEVELOPMENT, AND TRANSLATION[1]

---

[1] The National Academies of Sciences, Engineering, and Medicine's forums and roundtables do not issue, review, or approve individual documents. The responsibility for the published Proceedings of a Workshop rests with the workshop rapporteurs and the institution.

Forum Staff

CAROLYN SHORE, Forum Director
AMANDA WAGNER GEE, Program Officer
JENNIFER HINNERS, Program Officer
SYLVIA NCHA, Associate Program Officer
EESHAN KHANDEKAR, Associate Program Officer
MELVIN JOPPY, Senior Program Assistant
ANDREW M. POPE, Senior Director, Board on Health Sciences Policy

FORUM ON NEUROSCIENCE AND NERVOUS SYSTEM DISORDERS

FRANCES JENSEN (*Co-Chair*), University of Pennsylvania
JOHN KRYSTAL (*Co-Chair*), Yale University
SUSAN AMARA, Society for Neuroscience
RITA BALICE-GORDON, Sanofi
KATJA BROSE, Chan Zuckerberg Initiative
EMERY BROWN, Harvard Medical School and Massachusetts Institute of Technology
DANIEL BURCH, Pharmaceutical Product Development, LLC
JOSEPH BUXBAUM, Icahn School of Medicine at Mount Sinai
SARAH CADDICK, Gatsby Charitable Foundation
ROSA CANET-AVILÉS, Foundation for the National Institutes of Health
MARIA CARRILLO, Alzheimer's Association
EDWARD CHANG, University of California, San Francisco
TIMOTHY COETZEE, National Multiple Sclerosis Society
JONATHAN COHEN, Princeton University
ROBERT CONLEY, Eli Lilly and Company
JAMES DESHLER, National Science Foundation
BILLY DUNN, U.S. Food and Drug Administration
MICHAEL EGAN, Merck Research Laboratories
NITA FARAHANY, Duke University School of Law
JOSHUA GORDON, National Institute of Mental Health
RAQUEL GUR, University of Pennsylvania
MAGALI HAAS, Cohen Veterans Bioscience
RAMONA HICKS, One Mind
RICHARD HODES, National Institute on Aging
STUART HOFFMAN, Department of Veterans Affairs
JONATHAN HORSFORD, National Institute of Dental and Craniofacial Research
YASMIN HURD, Icahn School of Medicine at Mount Sinai
STEVEN HYMAN, Broad Institute of Massachusetts Institute of Technology and Harvard University
MICHAEL IRIZARRY, Eisai Inc.
GEORGE KOOB, National Institute on Alcohol Abuse and Alcoholism
WALTER KOROSHETZ, National Institute of Neurological Disorders and Stroke
STORY LANDIS, National Institute of Neurological Disorders and Stroke (*Emeritus*)
ALAN LESHNER, American Association for the Advancement of Science (*Emeritus*)
HUSSEINI MANJI, Janssen Research & Development, LLC

CAROLINE MONTOJO, The Kavli Foundation
STEVEN PAUL, Voyager Therapeutics
EMILIANGELO RATTI, Takeda Pharmaceuticals International
TODD SHERER, The Michael J. Fox Foundation for Parkinson's Research
DAVID SHURTLEFF, National Center for Complementary and Integrative Health
SANTA TUMMINIA, National Eye Institute
NORA VOLKOW, National Institute on Drug Abuse
ANDREW WELCHMAN, Wellcome Trust
DOUG WILLIAMSON, Lundbeck
STEVIN ZORN, MindImmune Therapeutics, Inc.

Forum Staff

CLARE STROUD, Forum Director
SHEENA M. POSEY NORRIS, Program Officer
PHOENIX WILSON, Senior Program Assistant
ANDREW M. POPE, Senior Director, Board on Health Sciences Policy

NATIONAL CANCER POLICY FORUM

RICHARD L. SCHILSKY, American Society of Clinical Oncology
DEBORAH SCHRAG, Harvard Medical School and Dana-Farber Cancer Institute
LAWRENCE N. SHULMAN, University of Pennsylvania
DAN THEODORESCU, Cedars-Sinai Medical Center
GEORGE J. WEINER, The University of Iowa
ROBERT A. WINN, Virginia Commonwealth University

Forum Staff

ERIN BALOGH, Senior Program Officer
EMILY ZEVON, Associate Program Officer
KATE HAWTHORNE, Senior Program Assistant
ANNALEE GONZALES, Administrative Assistant
SHARYL NASS, Director, National Cancer Policy Forum, and Director, Board on Health Care Services

ROUNDTABLE ON GENOMICS AND PRECISION HEALTH

KAREN WECK, College of American Pathologists
CATHERINE WICKLUND, National Society of Genetic Counselors
HUNTINGTON F. WILLARD, Geisinger National Precision Health
JANET WILLIAMS, American Academy of Nursing
SARAH WORDSWORTH, University of Oxford

Roundtable Staff

SARAH BEACHY, Roundtable Director
SIOBHAN ADDIE, Program Officer
MEREDITH HACKMANN, Associate Program Officer
MICHAEL BERRIOS, Senior Program Assistant
ANDREW M. POPE, Senior Director, Board on Health Sciences Policy

Reviewers

This Proceedings of a Workshop was reviewed in draft form by individuals chosen for their diverse perspectives and technical expertise. The purpose of this independent review is to provide candid and critical comments that will assist the National Academies of Sciences, Engineering, and Medicine in making each published proceedings as sound as possible and to ensure that it meets the institutional standards for quality, objectivity, evidence, and responsiveness to the charge. The review comments and draft manuscript remain confidential to protect the integrity of the process.

We thank the following individuals for their review of this proceedings:

YARIMAR CARRASQUILLO, National Center for Complementary and Integrative Health, National Institutes of Health
ASHLEY FARLEY, Bill & Melinda Gates Foundation
RICHARD SEVER, Cold Spring Harbor Laboratory Press
GEETA K. SWAMY, Duke University

Although the reviewers listed above provided many constructive comments and suggestions, they were not asked to endorse the content of the proceedings nor did they see the final draft before its release. The review of this proceedings was overseen by **CAROLE LEE,** University of Washington. She was responsible for making certain that an independent examination of this proceedings was carried out in accordance with standards of the National Academies and that all review comments were carefully considered. Responsibility for the final content rests entirely with the rapporteurs and the National Academies.

Acknowledgments

Sponsorship from the Cell Press, *The Lancet*, the National Institutes of Health's Office of Extramural Research and Office of Science Policy, and Nature Research made this workshop—and the fruitful discussions therein—possible. Support from the many annual sponsors of the National Academies of Sciences, Engineering, and Medicine's Forum on Drug Discovery, Development, and Translation; Forum on Neuroscience and Nervous System Disorders; National Cancer Policy Forum; and Roundtable on Genomics and Precision Health is crucial to support this and other work of the National Academies.

The National Academies staff wish to express their gratitude to the speakers whose presentations helped inform workshop discussions on the state of transparent reporting in preclinical biomedical research; the members of the planning committee for their work in developing the workshop agenda and shaping the discussions; and the many other National Academies staff without whom this workshop and the accounting thereof would not have been possible: Jeanay Butler, Daniel Cesnalis, Robert Day, Sadaf Faraz, Greta Gorman, Anna Camilo Javier, Bardia Massoudkhan, Bettina Seliber, Lauren Shern, and Taryn Young.

Contents

Acronyms and Abbreviations

AlzPED	Alzheimer's Disease Preclinical Efficacy Database
ARRIVE	Animal Research: Reporting of In Vivo Experiments
CEO	chief executive officer
CONSORT	Consolidated Standards of Reporting Trials
COPE	Committee on Publication Ethics
CRO	clinical research organization
CTSA	Clinical and Translational Science Awards
ECNP	European College of Neuropsychopharmacology
EQIPD	European Quality in Preclinical Data
EQUATOR	Enhancing the QUAlity and Transparency Of health Research
FSU	Florida State University
ICMJE	International Committee of Medical Journal Editors
IRB	Institutional Review Board
JoVE	*Journal of Visualized Experiments*
MD	Standards for Preventing and Handling Missing Data
MDAR	materials, design, analysis, and reporting
METRICS	Meta-Research Innovation Center at Stanford University

NAS	National Academy of Sciences
NC3Rs	National Centre for the Replacement, Refinement and Reduction of Animals in Research
NCCIH	National Center for Complementary and Integrative Health (NIH)
NIH	National Institutes of Health (Department of Health and Human Services)
NINDS	National Institute of Neurological Disorders and Stroke (NIH)
NPQIP	Nature Publishing Group Quality in Publication
ORI	Office of Research Integrity
PCORI	Patient-Centered Outcomes Research Institute
PLOS	Public Library of Science
PRISMA	Preferred Reporting Items for Systematic Reviews and Meta-Analyses
PTSD	posttraumatic stress disorder
RCR	responsible conduct of research
RQR	rigor, quality, and reproducibility
SEPTRE	SPIRIT Electronic Protocol Tool and Resource
SPIRIT	Standard Protocol Items: Recommendations for Interventional Trials
STEM	science, technology, engineering, and mathematics
TOP	Transparency and Openness Promotion

1

Introduction[1]

Sharing knowledge is what drives scientific progress—each new advance or innovation in biomedical research builds on previous observations. However, for experimental findings to be broadly accepted as credible by the scientific community, they must be verified by other researchers. An essential step is for researchers to report their findings in a manner that is understandable to others in the scientific community and provide sufficient information for others to validate the original results and build on them.

In recent years, concern has been growing over a number of studies that have failed to replicate previous results and evidence from larger meta-analyses, which have pointed to the lack of reproducibility in biomedical research (e.g., Bik et al., 2016, 2018; Ioannidis, 2005; Landis et al., 2012; Sena et al., 2010). In response, funders, publishers, and other key stakeholders have recognized the need to encourage and enhance transparent reporting of preclinical research findings across the biomedical research life cycle (e.g., Kiley et al., 2017; McNutt, 2014; Nosek et al.,

[1] This workshop was organized by an independent planning committee whose role was limited to identification of topics and speakers. This Proceedings of a Workshop was prepared by the rapporteurs as a factual summary of the presentations and discussion that took place at the workshop. Statements, recommendations, and opinions expressed are those of individual presenters and participants and are not endorsed or verified by the National Academies of Sciences, Engineering, and Medicine, and they should not be construed as reflecting any group consensus.

2015; the Center for Open Science;[2] policies at the National Institutes of Health [NIH],[3] the Gates Foundation,[4] or the Wellcome Trust;[5] or broadly accepted policy statements such as in the case of public health emergencies[6]). On September 25 and 26, 2019, the National Academies of Sciences, Engineering, and Medicine (the National Academies) hosted a public workshop in Washington, DC, to discuss the current state of transparency in the reporting of preclinical biomedical research and to explore opportunities for harmonizing reporting guidelines across journals and funding agencies. The workshop primarily focused on transparent reporting in preclinical research, but also considered lessons learned and best practices from clinical research reporting. The agenda for the workshop, titled Enhancing Scientific Reproducibility in Biomedical Research Through Transparent Reporting, was developed by an independent planning committee; the workshop Statement of Task is available in Box 1-1.[7] The workshop was convened jointly by the Forum on Drug Discovery, Development, and Translation; the Forum on Neuroscience and Nervous System Disorders; the National Cancer Policy Forum; and the Roundtable on Genomics and Precision Health, and was sponsored by the Cell Press, *The Lancet*, the National Institutes of Health, and Nature Research.

This workshop builds on recent consensus reports by the National Academies, including *Reproducibility and Replicability in Science* (NASEM, 2019, discussed further in Chapter 2), *Open Science by Design: Realizing a Vision for 21st Century Research* (NASEM, 2018), and *Fostering Integrity in Research* (NASEM, 2017). Selected guidelines and checklists for transparent reporting were also discussed and brief background information was provided to participants to facilitate the discussions (available in Appendix B).

---

[2] See https://cos.io (accessed January 13, 2020).

[3] See https://grants.nih.gov/policy/reproducibility/index.htm (accessed January 10, 2020).

[4] Open access policy available at https://www.gatesfoundation.org/How-We-Work/General-Information/Open-Access-Policy (accessed January 13, 2020).

[5] Open research policies available at https://wellcome.ac.uk/what-we-do/our-work/open-research (accessed January 13, 2020).

[6] For more information, see https://wellcome.ac.uk/press-release/statement-data-sharing-public-health-emergencies (accessed February 10, 2020).

[7] The workshop agenda can be found in Appendix C. Archived webcast videos and speakers' presentations are available on the National Academies website. See http://nationalacademies.org/hmd/Activities/Research/DrugForum/2019-Sept-25.aspx (accessed November 20, 2019).

BOX 1-1
Workshop Statement of Task

An ad hoc committee of the National Academies of Sciences, Engineering, and Medicine will plan and conduct a public workshop to discuss the current state of transparency in reporting biomedical research (e.g., disclosure of the availability and location of data, materials, analysis, and methodology) and to explore the possibility of improving the harmonization of guidelines across journals and funding agencies so that biomedical researchers propose and report data in a consistent manner.

Workshop objectives:

- Highlight current efforts by researchers, institutions, funders, and journals to increase transparency in proposing and reporting preclinical biomedical research;
- Discuss journal and funder assessments of researchers' adherence to reporting guidelines, including a discussion of the effectiveness of checklists;
- Consider lessons learned from field-specific best practices for increased transparency in reporting rigor elements (research design, methodology, analysis, interpretation, reporting of results) that are generalizable across biomedical research domains;
- Discuss opportunities for improving the consistency of reporting guidelines and requirements for rigor and transparency by journals, funders, and institutions across the biomedical research life cycle; and
- Consider approaches to compare reporting of rigor elements proposed in grant applications to those included in publications.

The committee will plan and organize the workshop, develop the agenda, select and invite speakers and discussants, and moderate or identify moderators for the discussions. The agenda will include a panel discussion on facilitating the development of consistent guidelines (e.g., a common set of minimal reporting standards) that could be applied across journals and funders to increase transparency in proposing and reporting biomedical research. Proceedings of the presentations and discussions at the workshop will be prepared by a designated rapporteur in accordance with institutional guidelines.

ORGANIZATION OF THE PROCEEDINGS

This Proceedings of a Workshop summarizes the presentations and discussions that took place at the workshop. As background for the workshop discussions, an overview of the findings and recommendations of the most recent National Academies consensus study related to reproducibility in scientific research, *Reproducibility and Replicability in Science*, was presented by Harvey Fineberg, president of the Gordon and Betty Moore Foundation and chair of both the workshop and the consensus study

(Chapter 2). Participants were also addressed by National Academy of Sciences (NAS) President Marcia McNutt, who delivered a keynote talk on sustaining public trust in science (Chapter 2). The first workshop panel focused on the current culture of science as it relates to transparency in proposing and reporting preclinical biomedical research. Researchers representing different roles in the science ecosystem shared their perspectives on the incentives, disincentives, challenges, and opportunities associated with transparent reporting and replicability in science (Chapter 3). The second panel considered lessons learned and best practices for increased transparency from the field of clinical research that could be applied to improving transparent reporting of preclinical studies (Chapter 4). In the third panel session, speakers explored the practical application and effectiveness of checklists and guidelines for enhancing transparent reporting of biomedical research (Chapter 5). In the final panel session, speakers representing different stakeholders discussed opportunities for action to harmonize guidelines and develop a common set of minimal reporting standards (Chapter 6). The last session of the workshop provided an opportunity for all participants to engage in small group discussions to apply what they had learned throughout the workshop and consider what actions researchers, publishers, institutions, and funders could take to improve transparent reporting of biomedical research (Chapter 7). Points of interest were shared on Twitter throughout the workshop by participants using the hashtag #reproducibilityinscience.[8]

[8] The Twitter discussion that took place on September 25 and 26 in association with the workshop can be viewed at https://twitter.com/hashtag/ReproducibilityInScience (accessed November 20, 2019).

2

Transparency and Trust

To establish a foundation for the workshop discussions, Harvey Fineberg, president of the Gordon and Betty Moore Foundation and workshop chair, elaborated on the findings and recommendations of the recently published National Academies of Sciences, Engineering, and Medicine report *Reproducibility and Replicability in Science* (NASEM, 2019). Marcia McNutt, president of the National Academy of Sciences (NAS) and former editor-in-chief of *Science*, delivered a keynote address to participants on signaling "indicators of trust" to the scientific community and the public.

OVERVIEW OF ***REPRODUCIBILITY AND REPLICABILITY IN SCIENCE***

Harvey Fineberg, President, Gordon and Betty Moore Foundation

The National Academies consensus study report *Reproducibility and Replicability in Science* was sponsored by the National Science Foundation.[1] The committee assessed research and data reproducibility issues with a focus on topics that cross disciplines. More specifically, the committee was charged with defining the terms "reproducibility" and "replicability" (see Box 2-1), examining the extent and impact of the lack of reproducibility

[1] The full report and additional information are available at https://sites.nationalacademies.org/sites/reproducibility-in-science/index.htm (accessed November 20, 2019).

BOX 2-1
Defining Reproducibility and Replicability

The committee found that different scientific fields use terminology differently, and even in contradictory ways. For the purposes of this report, the committee defined the terms as follows:

- "*Reproducibility* is obtaining consistent results using the same input data, computational steps, methods, and code, and conditions of analysis. This definition is synonymous with computational reproducibility" (NASEM, 2019, p. 36).
- "*Replicability* is obtaining consistent results across studies aimed at answering the same scientific question, each of which has obtained its own data" (NASEM, 2019, p. 36).

While reproducibility is often used by the National Institutes of Health and others to encompass both the computational and replication aspects of a scientific experiment, Fineberg said the committee believed it was important to distinguish between them because the consequences of failure to computationally reproduce or to replicate can be very different. For the purposes of this workshop, however, the discussions of enhancing scientific reproducibility encompass both aspects (i.e., transparent reporting has implications for both computational reproduction and replication, as they were defined by the consensus committee in its report).

SOURCE: Fineberg presentation, September 25, 2019.

and replicability on the overall health of science and engineering, and reviewing current activities to improve reproducibility and replicability.

The main conclusion of the study, Fineberg summarized, is that there is no "crisis" with regard to replication and reproducibility of scientific findings, "but there is also no room for complacency." "Reproducibility is critically important," he continued, but is "not currently easy to attain." The committee noted their concerns about the non-replicability of individual studies. Furthermore, the report states that neither reproducibility nor replicability alone can ensure the reliability of scientific knowledge.

Reproducibility

A challenge for computational reproducibility across scientific disciplines is that many reports of studies do not include sufficient information to allow another researcher to reproduce the original computational results, Fineberg said. The committee found that less than half of the studies they reviewed provided the "full array of data, code, digital artifacts, and other elements required" to facilitate computational reproducibility.[2] There is growing recognition of this problem, Fineberg acknowledged. He shared several examples of efforts to provide more complete data and information (e.g., providing Internet links to underlying datasets and code, marking articles with badges that indicate open data sharing).

The committee identified several obstacles to reproducibility, Fineberg reported, including inadequate recordkeeping, reporting that lacks critical elements, obsolete digital artifacts, errors in the attempts to reproduce the findings of others, and cultural barriers.[3] The committee also noted that improving computational reproducibility is challenging because experiments are complex and involve multiple steps that must be systematically documented and reported. In some cases, full reproducibility is not possible as studies involve non-public or proprietary data and experimental components.

Replicability

As defined by the committee, replicability is nuanced and complex, especially with regard to the implications of failure to replicate. "Replicability takes many forms," Fineberg said, and some studies are inherently not replicable (e.g., studies of ephemeral phenomena such as an earthquake; long-term epidemiological studies). The committee also observed that many studies are replicated as part of the routine conduct of science and these replications are not reported because the intent is to reaffirm a previous finding in order to build on it.

The committee outlined several situations in which undertaking the replication of a particular study might be necessary or appropriate. Fineberg listed several examples: if the results of the original study are to be used in making decisions of consequence (e.g., policy, clinical, or investment decisions); if the original study produced controversial or unexpected results; if the original study is flawed (e.g., design, methods, analysis); or if "the costs of replication are offset by the potential benefits for science and society." Some studies are more replicable than others, and the committee's report discusses the contributing roles of the complexity of the system under study and the degree of experimental control that is

[2] See Table 4-1 in NASEM (2019) for studies that have assessed computational reproducibility.

[3] For detailed discussion, see pp. 55–58 in NASEM (2019).

possible. The lower the complexity and the higher the controllability, the better the chance of replication, Fineberg explained.[4]

The committee concluded that "the occurrence of non-replicability is due to multiple sources, some of which impede and others of which promote progress in science" (NASEM, 2019, p. 85). The committee differentiated between sources of non-replicability that are "potentially helpful" and those that are "unhelpful" to the advancement of science. A helpful reason for non-replicability of a study, for example, could be the identification of a new natural source of variability or other new discovery. Unhelpful, and potentially avoidable, sources of non-replicability include simple mistakes, methodological errors, bias, and fraud. Another unhelpful source of non-replicability discussed by the committee was inappropriate statistical inference, and Fineberg noted the problem of "misunderstanding and misuse of the concepts of *p*-values and statistical significance."[5] Efforts are being made to address these unhelpful sources of non-replicability, he continued, such as the development of guidelines and checklists for researchers and other approaches to increase awareness and improve reporting and transparency.

Workshop Participant Comments on Replicability

Workshop participants shared several examples how failure to replicate led to new insights. Thomas Curran, executive director and chief scientific officer of Children's Mercy, Kansas City, observed that errors in replicability can lead to new discoveries. He shared an example in which the majority of published research describing a new cancer drug target was wrong due to the use of an inappropriate model, but further research revealed the applicability of the target to rare cancers and led to new drugs that might not otherwise have been developed. Another participant shared that variability in the replicability of a study he had published was ultimately associated with the amount of time the samples were exposed to oxygen during handling. It took years to figure out that the sample was easily oxidized, and those who handled samples anaerobically could replicate the experiment while others could not.

Participants also commented on statistics in replicability. John Gardenier, a research ethicist, agreed with the concerns raised by the committee about statistical analysis and reliance on *p*-values. He noted that the use of *p*-values is considered "standard in science," but that does not necessarily make it appropriate or ethical. Kay Lund, director of the Division

---

[4] For further discussion, see Figure 5-2 on p. 74 in NASEM (2019).
[5] See pp. 75–85 and Appendix D in NASEM (2019).

of Biomedical Research Workforce at the National Institutes of Health, expressed concern about underpowered animal studies that are carried out in response to peer review or to meet criteria for publication.[6] She noted that there is generally no mention in the publication that these add-on studies are preliminary data.

Public Trust in Science

The consensus committee reviewed data on public trust in science, Fineberg continued, and found that, from 1978 to 2018, the level of public confidence in the scientific community has been consistently higher than public confidence in other institutions, including major companies, the press, and Congress. Only the military has garnered higher public trust in recent decades, he said.[7]

Recommendations from the Consensus Study Report *Reproducibility and Replicability in Science*

Following its assessment of reproducibility and replicability in science, the committee made numerous recommendations directed toward funders, policy makers, researchers, journal editors and publishers, conference organizers, educational institutions, professional societies, and journalists. Fineberg highlighted four of the committee's recommendations as being particularly relevant for the workshop discussions (see Box 2-2). These address the need for researchers to report complete information, and the roles that various stakeholders play—including academic institutions, professional societies, researchers, funders, and journals—in increasing transparency in the reporting of science for the purpose of enhancing scientific reproducibility and replicability.

In closing, Fineberg summarized that data sharing and transparent reporting should be an expectation of the scientific community. Barriers to the persistent availability of the digital artifacts and reagents needed for reproducibility and replicability include costs, lack of infrastructure, the culture of science, and weak incentives, he said. "There is a great deal that has already been accomplished," he said, and he encouraged workshop participants to consider how existing principles and practices can be endorsed, leveraged, or improved upon to further the progress toward transparency in science.

---

[6] Discussed further by Vinson and others in Chapter 6.
[7] For detailed discussion, see p. 127 in NASEM (2019).

BOX 2-2
Select Report Recommendations Relevant to the Workshop

RECOMMENDATION 6-1: "All researchers should include a clear, specific, and complete description of how the reported result was reached. Different areas of study or types of inquiry may require different kinds of information."

RECOMMENDATION 6-6: "Many stakeholders have a role to play in improving computational reproducibility, including educational institutions, professional societies, researchers, and funders.

- Educational institutions should educate and train students and faculty about computational methods and tools....
- Professional societies should take responsibility for educating the public and their professional members about ... computational research ... [and] the evolving nature of science....
- Researchers should collaborate with expert colleagues....
- [Funders] should consider funding of activities to promote computational reproducibility."

RECOMMENDATION 6-7: "Journals and scientific societies requesting submissions for conferences should disclose their policies relevant to achieving reproducibility and replicability.... Journals and conference organizers are encouraged to:

- Set and implement desired standards of reproducibility and replicability and make this one of their priorities, such as deciding which level they wish to achieve for each Transparency and Openness Promotion guideline and working towards that goal;
- Adopt policies to reduce the likelihood of non-replicability, such as considering incentives or requirements for research materials transparency, design, and analysis plan transparency, enhanced review of statistical methods, study or analysis plan preregistration, and replication studies; and
- Require as a review criterion that all research reports include a thoughtful discussion of the uncertainty in measurements and conclusions."

RECOMMENDATION 6-9: "Funders should require a thoughtful discussion in grant applications of how uncertainties will be evaluated, along with any relevant issues regarding replicability and computational reproducibility. Funders should introduce review of reproducibility and replicability guidelines and activities into their merit-review criteria, as a low-cost way to enhance both."

NOTE: Recommendation numbers refer to the numbering scheme used in the report.
SOURCES: Fineberg presentation, September 25, 2019; adapted from NASEM, 2019, pp. 89, 103, 111, and 116, respectively.

SUSTAINING PUBLIC TRUST IN SCIENCE

Marcia McNutt, President, National Academy of Sciences

McNutt opened her keynote address with a recent case example published in *The Chronicle of Higher Education* that illustrates the importance of research transparency.[8] As summarized by McNutt, the case, from the field of criminology, involved an anonymous whistleblower who found statistical irregularities in five published papers and emailed his concerns to all of the co-authors of each of the papers. One co-author, a faculty member at Florida State University (FSU), was listed on all five papers and held all the data. All the other co-authors responded that they had not seen the data. A co-author who was an associate professor at a university in New York followed up on the whistleblower's concerns because the FSU faculty member was his former mentor. The associate professor contacted his mentor to get the original data with the intention of helping to sort out any mistakes and protect his mentor's reputation. However, McNutt said the mentor did not provide the complete data.

The data in question involved phone surveys to landline phone numbers. As the assistant professor started to investigate, he observed that the response rate reported in the paper was more than 60 percent, which is well out of line with current response rates for such surveys. In addition, McNutt summarized from the article that the entity that conducted the survey was not identified, no source of funding was noted, and missing survey values had been filled in with imputed values.

The associate professor then sent a letter to the journal *Criminology*, which had published the paper on which he was a co-author. He also posted the letter online, which led to coverage of the case by Retraction Watch. The lead author of that paper then became involved and sought to retract the paper or correct it. McNutt read quotes from *The Chronicle Review* article, which suggested that the editor-in-chief of *Criminology*, who happened to be a university colleague of the associate professor, was highly resistant to a retraction despite the concerns raised by two co-authors of the paper. The quotes suggested that the editor was primarily concerned about the potential legal ramifications, impact on the mentor's reputation, and public relations that would result from a retraction, rather than the underlying issues with research quality. Furthermore, the comments by the editor indicated that he was aware that other papers published in his journal had been of questionable quality, but that he believed it was sufficient to simply alert the field, not retract publications.

[8] See https://www.chronicle.com/interactives/20190924-Criminology (accessed November 20, 2019).

Signaling Indicators of Trust

The case described in *The Chronicle Review* illustrates some of the key elements of transparency that are the focus of this workshop, including data availability, transparency of methods and statistics, and disclosure of funding sources. Another important aspect highlighted by this case, McNutt said, is the need to signal "indicators of trust" to the scientific community and the public. She said she found the response, or lack thereof, by the editor-in-chief of the journal to be particularly concerning. Not retracting the paper seemed acceptable to the editor because those in the field would know the work was problematic. The editor did not seem to care that other readers of the paper, including researchers outside that field of study, policy makers, and the general public, would not know the paper been discredited.

McNutt and colleagues recently addressed the issue of indicators of trust in a paper titled "Signaling the Trustworthiness of Science" (Jamieson et al., 2019). Three qualities that foster trust in the scientific enterprise are "competence, integrity, and benevolence," McNutt said. The norms of science promote these qualities, she continued, but scientists often do not "clearly signal" to others in the scientific community or to the public that these norms have been upheld, or when appropriate, that they have been violated.

A benefit of communicating the adherence to scientific norms is that it reinforces those norms in the community. McNutt mentioned the use of open science badges by journals as an example of signaling adherence to norms in published research. Badges, such as those developed by the Center for Open Science to indicate open data, open materials, and preregistration of research, are "self-reinforcing," she said. In the future, badges might also be displayed by journals for studies that have been independently reproduced or replicated, that have had independent statistics review, or that have been screened for plagiarism or image manipulation, she suggested. She noted that digital publishing of journals facilitates the display of additional badges after publication as appropriate.

A survey referred to by McNutt and colleagues found that the public places value on indicators of the trustworthiness of science. For example, respondents said "they are more likely to trust a study if scientists make data and methods transparent, if they disclose who funded the study, and if it is published in a peer-reviewed journal," she summarized (see Jamieson et al., 2019).

Improving Indicators of Trustworthiness

McNutt highlighted several areas in need of improvement that were discussed in Jamieson et al. (2019). One area is the need to improve the quality and transparency of the peer-review process. "Standards of peer review vary greatly among journals," she said, and "there are very few signals of quality of peer review." There are also cases in which journals have claimed they conduct peer review but do not, and cases of reviewer fraud.

Another area for attention is the language used for signaling the removal of a paper from the literature. McNutt pointed out that "retraction" is used to describe all withdrawals, whether due to honest errors or to falsification and fabrication, casting a negative light on all authors. The paper discusses the need for more descriptive terminology that signals the reason for removal of the paper from the literature. McNutt added that less punitive language could encourage more authors to withdraw their papers when errors are discovered.

As indicated by the survey, the public values information about potential biases. In this regard, McNutt said that "full disclosure of funding sources, outside obligations, and competing interests" is essential. Although journals generally require disclosures, she said more clarity is needed about what must be disclosed and for what time period. For example, for how long are past relationships relevant, or when do impending future relationships need to be disclosed? In addition, she said it is challenging for reviewers and editors to verify the accuracy of author disclosures.

In closing, McNutt expressed dismay that "members of the public are misled by long discredited studies," and she cited an infamous example of a discredited study on vaccines and autism that took a decade to retract after it was widely known in the field that the work was fraudulent. She emphasized that the scientific community must take action to send "consistent and meaningful signals of which studies are honoring the norms that sustain trust."

Discussion

Following the keynote presentation, participants raised several issues for discussion with McNutt.

Coordinating Across Sectors

A participant asked how more cross-sector coordination could be encouraged. McNutt suggested that one possibility could be to develop an ongoing National Academies forum to share best practices for integrity, trust, and transparency and coordinate action across stakeholder groups at the research enterprise level. She noted that different stakeholder groups have created their own entities, such as the Committee on

Publication Ethics (COPE) for publishers, but no function exists to help coordinate the activities across all phases of research "from funding to execution to publication."

Dealing with Misconduct[9]

Frustration with the lack of consequences for misconduct was noted by a participant. McNutt said she was initially concerned that imposing sanctions on researchers could lead to overreaction and backfire—concerns may not be reported for fear of ruining someone's career. Now, however, she believes there is a need for action by the appropriate bodies and added that "no one should be untouchable." The appropriate body would be the researcher's employer, she said, but could also be a funder (e.g., in cases of fraud or misappropriation of funds) or a journal (when an author's actions violate journal rules).

Harold Sox, program director of peer review at the Patient-Centered Outcomes Research Institute (PCORI), raised concerns about "the practice of spin" (e.g., when authors play up a positive secondary outcome when the primary outcome is negative). He said this is "a milder form of scientific misconduct." He suggested that journal editors need to better address this and that standards are needed to help reviewers recognize hype that is not supported by data. McNutt agreed and said that most journal editors are volunteers and, in general, training for reviewers and editors is limited and may not sufficiently prepare them to address issues such as spin. She mentioned a recent survey carried out by a journal, which indicated that stakeholders would like more training opportunities for reviewers. She suggested that reviewer training could be discussed at scientific society meetings, and that students, early career researchers, and senior investigators could all provide feedback on what would be most helpful for such reviewer training.

Communicating Corrections in the Literature

Shai Silberberg, director for research quality at the National Institute of Neurological Disorders and Stroke (NINDS), noted his concern that researchers remain reluctant to alert editors to honest errors in their publications because of the potential negativity. He suggested finding a way to give credit to those who do come forward, perhaps on a "Correction

[9] A participant observed that issues of sexual harassment and bullying are now being discussed in the context of scientific misconduct. Although not germane to the discussion of reproducibility and transparent reporting, the need for codes of conduct that might address this type of misconduct was discussed briefly by participants.

Watch" blog akin to Retraction Watch. McNutt cautioned that some might game the system and publish with the intent of being the first to issue a correction. She added that retractions are relatively infrequent, making it difficult to pilot interventions and to understand what the unintended consequences are. Steven Goodman, professor of medicine and health research and policy and co-director of the Meta-Research Innovation Center (METRICS) at Stanford University, referred to a recent publication from METRICS that proposes new taxonomy for amendments to the published literature (Fanelli et al., 2018). Goodman and colleagues propose a list of terms that credit authors or journals as appropriate for making corrections. He added that comments on the proposal were gathered at a workshop attended by representatives from major journals, COPE, the National Library of Medicine, and others. Deborah Sweet, vice president of editorial at Cell Press, noted the difficulty in getting authors to retract papers. She mentioned that *Cell* has introduced an "Editorial Note" in which editors can discuss an investigation associated with a paper that was ultimately not retracted or corrected. This communicates the fact that an investigation was done, she said, even though it was decided that no action was needed.

3

Approaches to Cultivate Transparent Reporting in Biomedical Research

Highlights of Key Points Made by Individual Speakers

- Lack of transparency impacts the ability of researchers to replicate an experiment or to understand why it could not be replicated. (Carrasquillo, Wolinetz)
- Education about transparent reporting of biomedical research should be targeted toward early career faculty, postdoctoral fellows, graduate students, and undergraduates. (Carrasquillo)
- Investigators and trainees who are contributing toward a culture of transparency and reproducibility should be recognized and rewarded. (Carrasquillo)
- Tenure evaluation criteria should be restructured so that value is placed on an investigator's efforts toward reproducibility and transparency (e.g., consider the rigor of research studies or whether published findings have been replicated by others). (Carrasquillo)
- In the complex, decentralized ecosystem of scientific research, "all groups contribute to the incentives and reward structure and all are influenced by it." (Nosek)
- "This is not one entity's problem alone to solve." Stakeholders must work collectively to identify and address the cultural barriers to rigor, transparency, and replicability. (Wolinetz)

- Preprint publication prior to peer review can increase transparency and help identify errors and problematic images before publication. (Casadevall)
- The retracting of a paper should not be a career-ending phenomenon, but rather a part of the research process in which studies are repeated and the corrected data are then published. (Casadevall)

The first workshop panel focused on the current culture of science as it relates to transparency in proposing and reporting preclinical biomedical research (see Box 3-1 for corresponding workshop session objectives). Four researchers, each fulfilling different roles in the science ecosystem, shared their perspectives on the incentives, disincentives, challenges, and opportunities associated with transparent reporting and replicability in science.

Yarimar Carrasquillo, an investigator at the National Center for Complementary and Integrative Health (NCCIH) at the National Institutes of Health (NIH), shared her perspective as an early career researcher, describing the impact of non-replicability of published studies on setting up a new research program and achieving tenure. Brian Nosek, co-founder of the Center for Open Science, discussed the work of the center to effect behavioral change that better reflects the cultural norms in science and leads to greater openness and reproducibility of research. Arturo Casadevall, professor of molecular microbiology and immunol-

BOX 3-1
Workshop Session Objectives

- Highlight current efforts by researchers, institutions, funders, and journals to increase transparency in proposing and reporting preclinical biomedical research.
- Discuss the incentives, disincentives, challenges, and opportunities for researchers when it comes to transparent reporting of preclinical biomedical research (e.g., pressure to publish, institutional resources, training, funding).
- Discuss experience with implementation of policies to encourage transparent reporting across the biomedical research life cycle.
- Consider the role of stakeholders in supporting a cultural shift toward transparent reporting in preclinical biomedical research.

SOURCE: Workshop agenda (available in Appendix C), September 25, 2019.

ogy at Johns Hopkins University and editor-in-chief of *mBio*, discussed approaches to reduce errors in published papers from a publisher's perspective, including raising awareness of researchers, posting preprints, reviewer education about errors, and submission of original data to repositories. Carrie Wolinetz, acting chief of staff and associate director for Science Policy in the Office of the Director at NIH, described areas where NIH has been working to implement policies that enhance rigor, replicability, and transparency.

The session was moderated by Alexa McCray, professor of medicine at Harvard Medical School and chair of the National Academies of Sciences, Engineering, and Medicine consensus study committee that released the report *Open Science by Design* (NASEM, 2018). Researchers are generally not recognized or rewarded for making their data available, McCray observed. She highlighted the first recommendation from the report, which addressed overcoming cultural barriers:

> Research institutions should work to create a culture that actively supports Open Science by Design by better rewarding and supporting researchers engaged in open science practices. Research funders should provide explicit and consistent support for practices and approaches that facilitate this shift in culture and incentives. (NASEM, 2018, p. 7)

The consensus study report *Reproducibility and Replicability in Science* also discusses efforts to "foster a culture that values and rewards openness and transparency," she said, and describes "guidelines that promote openness, badges and prizes that recognize openness, changes in policies to ensure transparent reporting, new approaches to publishing results, and direct support for replication efforts" (NASEM, 2019, p. 104).

EARLY CAREER INVESTIGATOR PERSPECTIVE

Yarimar Carrasquillo, Investigator, National Center for Complementary and Integrative Health

Carrasquillo emphasized the importance of targeting younger investigators, not only early career faculty and researchers, but also undergraduate students, graduate students, and postdoctoral fellows, when working to raise awareness about the need for transparent reporting of biomedical research. Many of the issues directly affect new investigators, she said, who are under pressure to publish in high-impact journals and to report "flashy science" that, while interesting, is often not biologically relevant. Engaging emerging investigators could help to facilitate the cultural change needed.

Establishing a New Laboratory

Lack of transparency in the reporting of biomedical research affects all researchers, from students to senior investigators, but it presents a particular challenge for early career investigators who are starting a new laboratory. "The tenure clock starts ticking immediately," Carrasquillo said. New principal investigators are working to build their research program, and they rely heavily on the literature for the information needed to develop methods and establish models for their studies. Many new faculty members find they cannot replicate studies in the literature.

Carrasquillo said her own efforts to establish her research program on pain mechanisms were set back by the inability to replicate published studies on the affective component of pain. Replicating the previous findings took 2 years, she said, because much of the information reported about experimental conditions and analyses, for example, was incomplete. This lengthy setback was frustrating for the trainee who was working to replicate the previous findings, and it could negatively impact Carrasquillo when her program is evaluated. Tenure-track investigators often find themselves revising their research plans because they cannot replicate the original findings. The inability to replicate the prior studies also raises concerns about the validity of the animal models of affective behavior, which she said impacts the ability to translate findings to clinical research.

By contrast, there were other models and methods that Carrasquillo wanted to incorporate into her program that she said were easy to replicate because there were detailed methods papers available (some with videos), and other publications that included raw values and individual data points. Carrasquillo observed that detailed methods papers are underappreciated in general and are not valued as scientific contributions for tenure review. She suggested that promoting and committing to transparent reporting is not enough. Transparency as a behavior needs to be valued and rewarded in concrete ways.

The Tenure Process

The tenure process values the quantity of publications and the impact factors of the journals in which they are published, Carrasquillo said. She reiterated that methods papers are not considered impactful and do not often appear in high-impact journals unless they describe innovative new protocols. Rigor, reproducibility, and transparency are time consuming, she continued, and are not generally rewarded in the tenure or promotion processes. She suggested the need for a system of both rewards and penalties for reproducibility and transparency, or the lack of them. Another challenge for early career investigators is attracting trainees. "Trainees in your lab will compare themselves with trainees in other labs and will resist rigorous processes if proper rewards are not in place," she said. It should also be recognized that early career investigators have fewer resources and less administrative and technical support compared with established investigators. An early career investigator must often work with trainees individually to review all data and foster a culture of rigorous science and transparency. Again, she said, this takes time, and it should be acknowledged that the research may not progress as quickly as it might in laboratories that do not espouse rigor and transparency, and laboratories that promote rigorous science should be appropriately rewarded. It also takes longer to publish, which is a problem for early career investigators because of the value the tenure process places on volume and impact of publications.

In response to a question, Carrasquillo said she has received support from senior faculty, especially from her scientific director, who encouraged her to draft a paper describing her laboratory's inability to initially replicate findings previously described in the literature as well as the troubleshooting process required to finally replicate the findings. A paper discussing factors that affect the replicability of experiments and that are known to substantially vary between labs is essential to move the field forward, she added. Although some senior faculty are understanding of replicability challenges and supportive of rigor and quality, it is not clear if a tenure committee would reward high-quality research that resulted in fewer publications.

Creating a Culture Change

Carrasquillo offered the following solutions to help overcome some of the obstacles that early career investigators face:

- Restructure tenure evaluation criteria so that efforts toward reproducibility and transparency are valued (e.g., methods papers, negative data). Consider the rigor of the studies conducted and whether the published findings have been replicated by others in the scientific community.
- Create a system of awards to recognize investigators and trainees who are contributing to a culture of transparency and reproducibility.

Carrasquillo also described how she has been working to promote a culture of reproducibility and transparency in her laboratory. Practices she has established in her laboratory include

- Meeting one on one with her trainees to ensure that experimental procedures are documented and reported in the methods section of publications;
- Recording detailed information about the materials used; and
- Requiring that experiments are performed blind and are replicated, from beginning to end, at least once or twice.

She noted several other practices that have been more challenging to implement, including labeling and organizing raw data so that they are easily accessible; getting trainees to accept that reporting data that do not align perfectly with their model is acceptable and is important for transparency; and having trainees document methods and analyses in real time so that details are not forgotten. She also observed that her field has not yet embraced preregistration of studies.

CULTURE CHANGE ORGANIZATION PERSPECTIVE

Brian Nosek, Co-Founder, Center for Open Science

The experiences described by Carrasquillo are not limited to early career researchers. Nosek described problems with replicability as "pervasive." As an example, he described the Replicability Project: Cancer Biology, a research project of the Center for Open Science. An analysis was done of the ability to replicate 197 experiments reported in 51 high-impact papers in preclinical cancer biology published from 2010 through 2012.[1] None of the 51 papers had all of the associated data available in a repository, Nosek said. A full dataset was readily available for just 3 of the 197 experiments described in the publications. Furthermore, none of the papers provided enough information to design a full protocol for any of the experiments. This emphasizes the core challenge of even having enough information to attempt a replication, he said.

Cultural Norms in Science

Nosek framed the cultural issues of replicability relative to Merton's norms of science and the associated counternorms (see Table 3-1). In addition to Merton's four original principles, Nosek added that quality versus quantity is another commonly expressed norm–counternorm.

The cultural challenge was illustrated by a survey of 3,300 early- and mid-career NIH awardees. Anderson and colleagues found that 90 percent of those surveyed endorsed the norms of science, and the major-

[1] For details, see https://osf.io/e81xl (accessed November 20, 2019).

TABLE 3-1 Norms and Counternorms in Science

Norms	Counternorms
Communality Open sharing of information with colleagues	Secrecy Closed, keeping information to oneself
Universalism Evaluate research on its own merit	Particularism Evaluate research by reputation/ past productivity of researcher
Disinterestedness Motivate by knowledge and discovery, not by personal gain	Self-interestedness Treat science as a competition with other scientists
Organized skepticism Consider all new evidence, even when it might contradict one's prior work or point of view	Organized dogmatism Invest career in promoting and defending one's own most important theories, findings, and innovations
Quality Seek quality contributions	Quantity Seek high volume

SOURCE: Nosek presentation, September 25, 2019.

ity of respondents also believed they personally behaved according to those norms (Anderson et al., 2007). However, the majority perceived the behavior of other scientists to be counternormative. In fact, Nosek explained, although scientists "collectively endorse the norms of science over the counternorms," the culture of science is "self-interested," with individuals focusing on advancing their own careers through "publishing in the right journals, presenting the right results, selectively reporting, and ignoring negative results."

Changing the Research Culture

Individual researchers, universities, publishers, funders, scientific societies, and other stakeholders populate the complex, decentralized ecosystem of scientific research. Nosek said that "all groups contribute to the incentives and reward structure and all are influenced by it." Coordination and cooperation are needed to bring about cultural change.

Nosek proposed a pyramid model for effecting cultural change and aligning researcher behavior with the values and norms that the scientific community espouses (see Figure 3-1). The necessary infrastructure to enable the desired behaviors forms the foundation of the pyramid. For successful adoption of behavioral change, that infrastructure should be accessible, easy to use, and adaptable to existing workflows. Making the

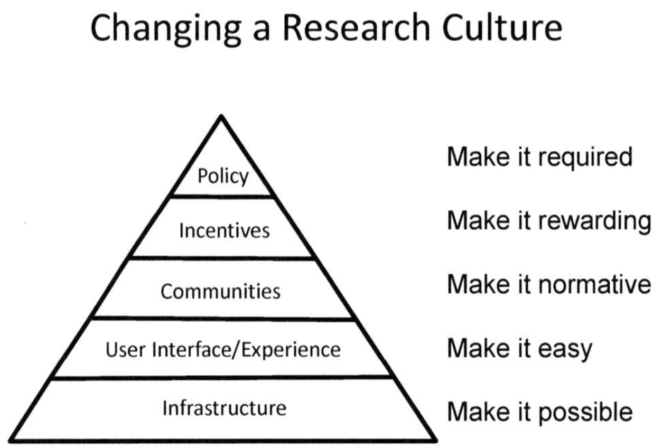

FIGURE 3-1 Pyramid model for effecting cultural change in science.
SOURCE: Nosek presentation, September 25, 2019.

desired behaviors visible in the scientific community encourages their adoption as norms. While some will readily conform to the new norms, others can be incentivized by rewards that align practically with their goals, Nosek continued. Some will not adapt their behavior unless it is mandated.

As an example, Nosek used preregistration of research as the desired behavior change. The infrastructure that makes preregistration possible includes project tools such as GitHub, Dropbox, Google Drive, Mendeley, and others. Integrating that infrastructure with other web applications, such as OSF Registries, helps to facilitate easy registration as part of routine workflow. Studies that conform to open science norms, such as preregistration, are awarded badges that make the practice visible in the community. Preregistration is now rewarded by more than 200 journals that are offering the Registered Reports publishing format as a submission option. Researchers submit their research plan to a journal for prestudy peer review. If the proposed study is accepted "in principle," it will be published upon completion regardless of outcome (assuming there are no issues with quality, clarity, or deviation from the registered plan). This means, Nosek explained, that the incentive is now on designing quality studies to answer important questions, not on getting positive results. Nosek reported that "about 60 percent of the articles that have been published so far through Registered Reports have negative results as their primary outcome," and these papers are cited as frequently as other articles. Finally, at the policy level, the Transparency and Openness Promotion (TOP) guidelines provide a framework for institutions, journals, and funders to use in implementing transparency standards.[2] Change is happening, Nosek said, and he shared data showing the increase from 38 preregistered studies in 2012 on OSF.io to a projected total of more than 35,000 in 2019. In response to a question, he clarified that the Registered Reports model specifically includes a commitment to publication as an incentive for preregistration, but other preregistration models are being used that do not use this incentive. Preregistration of research is broadly applicable to hypothesis testing and confirmatory experiments, he added.

Change needs to happen simultaneously, not sequentially, across all areas of the pyramid in Figure 3-1. Nosek said small communities (e.g., disease-specific funders) can have a large impact by changing their practices and then advocating to bring others into alignment.

SCIENTIFIC SOCIETY JOURNAL EDITOR PERSPECTIVE

Arturo Casadevall, Professor of Molecular Microbiology and Immunology, Johns Hopkins University, and Editor-in-Chief, mBio

Problematic figures and images are commonly found across the scientific literature. Casadevall said that "most problems are due to error, not misconduct, and new procedures are emerging to reduce error." To illustrate the extent of the problem, he described the findings of a systematic analysis initiated by Bik and colleagues (2016). The analysis involved visual inspection of more than 20,000 papers published in 39 journals across 13 publishers from 1995 to 2014. The study found problematic images in about 1 out of every 25 papers analyzed (about 4 percent). The prevalence of problematic images varied across different journals, and there was a steep increase in problematic images after the advent of photo editing software. These findings underestimate the prevalence, Casadevall said, because only photographic images were included in the analysis.

A second study analyzed 960 randomly selected papers that had been published in a single journal, *Molecular and Cellular Biology*, from 2009 to 2016 (Bik et al., 2018). This study found that more than 6 percent of images were problematic. Most of the problematic images identified were the result of errors, but 10 percent of the publications with problematic images were retracted. Based on the number of retractions, estimates showed that as many as 35,000 published papers could have images that

---

[2] Further information on the OSF Registries, Open Science Badges, Registered Reports, and TOP is available on the Center for Open Science website, https://cos.io (accessed November 20, 2019).

would prompt a retraction. Casadevall pointed out that finding and correcting problematic images in publications is costly and time intensive for journal staff, but increased image screening by journals prior to publication has led to a reduction in the number of these problematic images in published papers.

A similar analysis for errors was done of papers accepted for publication in the *Journal of Clinical Investigation* (Williams et al., 2019). Of the 200 papers analyzed, 28 percent were found to have "statistical issues" and 27 percent had problematic figures. Casadevall noted that the journal, of which he is a deputy editor, requires that authors submit copies of their original data when the paper is accepted for publication. When the problems with specific papers were investigated further, it was found that 89 percent were "minor transgressions," 7.5 percent were considered to be "moderate problems," and 1 percent of the papers had "major problems" that led the editors to rescind the acceptance.

In response to a question, Casadevall said that while the majority of retractions were due to misconduct, it is important to remember that retracted papers have multiple authors and the problems leading to retraction are often caused by a single author. Mechanisms are needed that do not stigmatize authors, but instead encourage retraction and allow for repeating of the studies and republication as appropriate.

Reducing Errors in Publications

An emerging option in biomedical publication is the ability to publicly post a preprint of the manuscript prior to peer review. Preprints increase transparency and allow researchers to rapidly share findings, but they can also help to catch errors before papers are published. Casadevall shared a personal example in which posting a preprint helped them to "avoid an embarrassing error." After posting, a reader noticed that one of the figures included a photo that had already been published. It was a simple error that was immediately corrected, Casadevall said. The number of preprints posted is increasing each year, and posted manuscripts are often revised based on feedback.

Casadevall described some of the emerging solutions to safeguard the literature (summarized in Box 3-2). In the prepublication phase, as discussed above, preprints allow other researchers in the field to both send comments directly to the authors and/or post them publicly in the preprint server. Increased education is making researchers aware that these types of errors are a problem and teaching them to check for errors before manuscripts are submitted. At the review and publication phases, reviewer education has led to reviewers looking at figures in manuscripts

BOX 3-2
Emerging Solutions to Safeguard the Literature

Prepublication Safeguards

- Public posting of preprints for presubmission feedback
- Increased education of researchers to raise awareness of the potential for errors in manuscripts
- Increased vigilance by researchers to check for errors in manuscripts

Review and Publication Safeguards

- Education of reviewers to enable more careful review of figures in manuscripts
- Enhanced editorial scrutiny of figures in submissions
- Requirements by journals for deposition of primary data into a repository

Post-Publication Safeguards

- Comments posted to websites such as PubPeer
- Comments submitted to journals regarding a recently published paper
- Reporting on publishing issues by the Retraction Watch website
- Retraction of a publication by the authors

SOURCE: Summarized from Casadevall presentation, September 25, 2019.

more carefully. There is also enhanced editorial scrutiny and requirements by some journals that the original data be submitted to the journal as a requirement for publication.

Errors identified by readers after publication are often disseminated on social media and websites such as PubPeer, Casadevall said, and there can be social media shaming. The blog Retraction Watch has exposed problems in many papers and investigates the reasons behind them. Comments are also submitted directly to journals. There are increasing numbers of retractions, and Casadevall said "scientists are beginning to realize the retracting of a paper is not a career-ending phenomenon." It should be a part of the research process; there are cases in which a paper is retracted, the studies are repeated, and the corrected data are then published.

Cultural aspects need to be addressed as well. Casadevall expressed concern, for example, that publishing a problematic paper in a high-impact journal is still better for one's career advancement than publishing a rigorous paper in a lower tier journal, and this is unacceptable, he said.

NATIONAL INSTITUTES OF HEALTH PERSPECTIVE

Carrie Wolinetz, Acting Chief of Staff and Associate Director for Science Policy, Office of the Director, National Institutes of Health

Wolinetz observed that rigor and transparency are sometimes considered to be barriers to scientific progress, and some believe that devoting resources to rigor and ensuring transparency takes resources away from research. NIH considers the tools of transparency to be essential components of science, not separate, she said, and resources should be spent on ensuring high-quality research. As a publicly funded research agency, NIH is accountable to the public, and transparency is a tool for demonstrating that NIH is a good steward of taxpayer dollars and is worthy of the public's trust. Wolinetz gave several examples of why transparency matters to scientists, the public, and research participants (see Box 3-3).

As a funder, NIH is in a position to influence policy and practice in science. However, "this is not one entity's problem alone to solve," Wolinetz said. Stakeholders must work collectively to identify and address the

BOX 3-3
Responsible Sharing of Information

Transparency matters to:

Scientists
- Raises the bar for ensuring rigorous research
- Maximizes investment by reducing unnecessary duplication
- Allows data and results to be combined in unconventional ways

The Public
- Acknowledges that publicly funded research is accountable to taxpayers
- Fosters greater public trust
- Facilitates better stewardship of research funds (less duplication of existing data, more advanced research)

Research Participants
- Brings research to the community
- Enables society to contribute to improving health
- Maximizes volunteer contribution
- Ensures the public is represented in research

SOURCE: Wolinetz presentation, September 25, 2019.

cultural barriers to rigor, transparency, and replicability in the scientific ecosystem. She observed that it is often assumed that "scientists know how to do science and are good at doing science and ... are equally good at training others how to do science." In reality, this is not necessarily true.

Reporting Clinical Trials Results

One area where NIH has been working to implement policies that enhance rigor, replicability, and transparency is the conduct of clinical trials, including the reporting of results (Hudson et al., 2016).[3] Transparency starts with the grant solicitation and spans the length of the clinical trial process, from initial study design through reporting of results, she said.

Responsible Data Sharing

Another area of focus for NIH is enabling and incentivizing responsible data sharing, Wolinetz said. In developing future policy in this area, NIH is looking to establish a flexible framework that "sets a floor for good practices" and enables the sharing of diverse types and amounts of data. Researchers seeking NIH funding will be required to provide a plan for how they intend to manage and share their data responsibly. Wolinetz said NIH is considering how plans for data management and sharing might be assessed as part of funding decisions, and how best to implement incentives and accountability measures to ensure commitments to sharing are met. She noted that there is a "push–pull relationship" in the pyramid discussed by Nosek (see Figure 3-1) in that the foundational infrastructure facilitates the implementation of policy, but development of that infrastructure is sometimes resisted until it is required by policy.

NIH released "Proposed Provisions for a Draft NIH Data Management and Sharing Policy" in 2018 to gather input that would inform the development of the draft policy. Wolinetz anticipated that a draft policy would be released for public comment in October 2019, with the intention of finalizing a policy in early 2020.[4] Angela Abitua, outreach scientist at Addgene, asked whether the forthcoming NIH policy on responsible data sharing will address the reporting and sharing of biological materials, such as plasmids, antibodies, and cell lines, which are used in the experiments. She observed that many journals have policies

---

[3] See also NIH Policy on the Dissemination of NIH-Funded Clinical Trial Information, https://grants.nih.gov/policy/clinical-trials/reporting/understanding/nih-policy.htm (accessed November 20, 2019).

[4] For current information, see https://osp.od.nih.gov/scientific-sharing/nih-data-management-and-sharing-activities-related-to-public-access-and-open-science (accessed November 20, 2019).

requiring the sharing of materials. Wolinetz said that biospecimens and other biological materials have been part of the discussions of sharing beyond data, specifically with respect to validation and sources of biological materials.

Rigor and Transparency

Wolinetz also discussed NIH's efforts to enhance rigor and reproducibility in biomedical research. She observed that the emphasis is beginning to move from reproducibility to transparency. Biology is complex and "biological experiments might not be reproducible," she said. Elucidating why an experiment could not be replicated could lead to a new discovery or a new research question. Transparency is essential to being able to replicate an experiment or to understand why it could not be replicated.

One current area of focus for NIH is rigor and reproducibility in animal research. Wolinetz pointed out that a large amount of NIH-funded research involves animal models, which she said are "incredibly important for advancing our understanding of biology and seeking new treatments for human diseases." Rigor in the design and conduct of experiments using animal models relates not only to designing appropriately powered experiments, but also to whether the animal model chosen is the best model to address the research question. Wolinetz noted that addressing rigor in animal research presents cultural challenges. In many cases, for example, a given animal model has been used by many researchers for many years, and there are numerous publications. Raising concerns that that model might not be appropriate to answer the questions asked or to model a particular human condition can meet resistance, and the subject-matter experts on that model have a vested interest in continuing to use it. A working group of the NIH Advisory Committee to the Director has been charged with considering rigor in animal research and making recommendations for improvement.[5]

DISCUSSION

Preserving Mertonian Norms in Science

Richard Sever, co-founder of bioRxiv and medRxiv and executive editor at the Cold Spring Harbor Laboratory Press, observed that the environment for early career investigators is more competitive than ever. The number of doctoral students continues to increase, but the number of

---

[5] See https://acd.od.nih.gov/working-groups/eprar.html (accessed November 20, 2019).

tenured faculty positions has remained steady. He suggested that the lack of job security may be related to the lack of willingness to be transparent with one's research and that "the academic career structure ... is now actively blocking transparency." Casadevall said students should be made aware that scientists are needed to fill many roles outside of academic tenure-track positions.

Sever also suggested that the obsession with publishing in high-impact journals is one of the causes of the culture shift from the norms of science toward the counternorms. The consequences of not publishing in high-impact journals are perceived as severe (e.g., unemployment). Casadevall said the impact factor obsession is widely acknowledged as a problem, but it persists because scientists are invested in the system. He suggested that nothing will change unless a large number of prominent scientists decide to take action. "The problem is sociological," he said. Valda Vinson, research editor at *Science*, added that impact factors were never intended to be used in this way (i.e., as a metric for hiring, tenure, or promotion).

McCray mentioned the Public Library of Science (PLOS) as an example of an initiative taken by scientists to improve openness and transparency. Casadevall described several examples of how he has been working to change these practices locally. As a department chair at Johns Hopkins, for example, he was able to change the hiring process for new faculty so that a curriculum vitae is not ranked by the impact factors of the papers listed. Rather, the content of the papers was considered, and applicants were selected for interviews based on the work described. Similarly, he and others were able to dissuade the tenure and promotions committee from requiring impact factors on a curriculum vitae. He described this as an ongoing battle that must be fought every day, by many people, on multiple levels before change will take hold. Casadevall and McCray encouraged participants to advocate for change in their departments and organizations. Goodman shared that Stanford is also moving away from counting publications and considering the journals they were published in for promotion review, and moving toward reading a sample of papers in depth for quality. The challenge of assessing quality instead of quantity, however, is reaching consensus on what constitutes quality, and how the quality of a candidate's publications can be assessed efficiently and consistently given that several individuals will each read one paper and write their analysis and recommendation. He observed that peer reviews of a given manuscript submitted for publication can vary widely. Casadevall agreed that robust mechanisms are needed and that methods to assess quality and rigor need to be studied.

Nosek suggested that, while changing the overall structure of publishing is a long-term goal, the focus now should be on incentivizing near-term behavioral changes. Scientists will continue to seek to publish in top-tier journals, he said. What can be changed is how those journals evaluate manuscripts for publication (e.g., implement requirements for rigor, transparency, preregistration) and how those publications are used by others, such as tenure committees (e.g., assess the quality of several papers rather than simply counting the number of publications in high-impact journals).

Facilitating Reproducibility

Jennifer Heimberg, senior program officer at the National Academies, pointed out that all publications in the *Journal of Visualized Experiments* (*JoVE*) include video recordings demonstrating the methods reported in the papers. In addition to increasing transparency, she said this approach allows for communication of nuances that might be missed in a written protocol. Casadevall noted that he has published in *JoVE* and Carrasquillo said that a *JoVE* paper contributed to the successful replication of a method by her laboratory, but both agreed that the weight of publications in *JoVE* and other journals of its type is lower than for publications in higher impact journals despite the valuable contribution of *JoVE* papers to replicability and training.

Guna Rajagopal, vice president of computational sciences, discovery science at Janssen R&D, shared that they and other pharmaceutical research programs often contact the authors of publications to discuss their studies and send company scientists to the authors' laboratories for several months to work together to address any issues and to reproduce the data, with support from the company. Unfortunately, the resulting information remains within the company due to intellectual property concerns. Casadevall acknowledged this concern and urged Rajagopal to find a way to share the information learned from these replication studies through peer-reviewed publications.

Correcting the Literature

Thomas Curran observed that, in his experience, high-impact journals are not interested in correcting the historical literature. Vinson emphasized that the integrity of the material a journal publishes is "the most important thing," and she supported efforts to change the metrics used for tenure and hiring decisions. She was very concerned about Curran's comment and was interested in being provided with examples. A challenge, she said, is that standards evolve, and the journal receives inquiries looking to apply a current standard to papers that were published prior to that standard being implemented. Another challenge is that, although journals do try to address concerns by negotiating corrections with authors, journals defer to the author's institution to conduct an investigation.

Calling Out Bad Behavior

Carrasquillo observed that early career investigators can be hesitant to call out bad science because it could earn them a reputation as a "troublemaker" and result in them not being asked by journals to review papers anymore, or even in retaliation by other scientists. Casadevall responded that journals value rigorous review, and investigators should not be worried about expressing their concerns about a manuscript. On the other hand, public criticism is often made without having all of the facts. He encouraged researchers to work within the system, gathering data on published errors, publishing them in peer-reviewed journals, and only then discussing the findings publicly, as was done with the analysis of figure problems he described. Wolinetz agreed that many people are hesitant to call out bad behavior by others because the culture in science places extremely high value on reputation. The *perception* that pointing out bad behavior leads to retaliation and has adverse effects on reputation is in and of itself a problem, because then just the perception is enough to drive behavior and reinforce a culture that is not desirable even if the reality is different, Wolinetz said. Carrasquillo agreed with Casadevall about the need to remove the stigma of "bad behavior" from retractions and for researchers not to take personal offense to errors being flagged.

Sustainability and Cost Considerations

Curran raised the issue of sustainability, noting that in some cases, volumes of data from NIH-supported data acquisition studies have become inaccessible after the end of the study due to a lack of funding at NIH to maintain the online database. Wolinetz agreed and said NIH is aware of these sustainability issues. This example demonstrates the importance of infrastructure and tools for data sharing and transparency. She emphasized that experimentation and infrastructure should not be pitted against each other when it comes to determining funding priorities.

Malcolm Macleod, professor at the University of Edinburgh, observed that there are many who call for improving the quality of science, but few who are prepared to invest the resources and commit to the extensive work that is required to ensure that quality. Simply increasing incentives will not cause the system to self-correct. Casadevall agreed and added that it is expensive for journals to hire staff to address these issues, and doing so could lead to higher journal publishing fees. Correcting errors after publication is even more expensive, he said.

Wolinetz added that the practical realities and downstream consequences of implementing any policy need to be recognized. "Are we willing to pay for the values that we are espousing, and what are the downstream consequences?" For example, to increase rigor, certain standards of statistical analysis could be enforced that would result in the need for more animals per study, which increases the cost per study. Given a fixed amount of funding to award, this results in an agency being able to fund fewer studies. She emphasized the need to think holistically and balance the trade-offs.

4

Lessons Learned and Best Practices

Highlights of Key Points Made by Individual Speakers

- Transparency in reporting begins with study design. Training in proper study design is needed for preclinical scientists. (Chan, Goodman, Kiermer)
- Rewards and incentives can inspire good behavior, but enforcement is also needed and is time and resource intensive. (Chan)
- Reporting guidelines should be promoted as beneficial and not burdensome for researchers. For example, submitting high-quality protocols facilitates more rapid Institutional Review Board review and leads to fewer queries and requests for revisions. (Chan)
- Funders have opportunities to influence and enable the rigor and reproducibility of studies they fund (e.g., providing feedback on proposals, tools and training, statistical support, and translational expertise; requiring data sharing for milestone payments; providing sufficient funding for data curation and management as well as open-access publication fees). (Haas)
- A research culture that promotes research integrity should be inclusive, comprehensive, multifaceted, pragmatic, and empowering. (Swamy)

As discussed by the first panel, transparent reporting of preclinical biomedical research is one element in the complex ecosystem of scientific research. Panelists discussed how the barriers to transparent reporting are rooted in the current culture of science and current incentive structures, and emphasized the importance of coordination across all stakeholders in fostering a culture of greater transparency. The second panel considered lessons learned and best practices for increased transparency from the field clinical research that could be applied to improving transparent reporting of preclinical studies (see Box 4-1 for corresponding workshop session objectives).

Veronique Kiermer, executive editor at the Public Library of Science and session moderator, mentioned the Consolidated Standards of Reporting Trials (CONSORT) guidelines as an example of an initiative to facilitate more complete reporting of randomized controlled trials.[1] The development of the CONSORT guidelines began in the mid-1990s, leading to the release of the first CONSORT Statement in 1996. Revised CONSORT Statements were released in 2001 and 2010. The International Committee of

BOX 4-1
Workshop Session Objectives

- Consider lessons learned from institutional and/or field-specific best practices for increased transparency in reporting rigor elements (i.e., research design, methodology, analysis, interpretation, and reporting of results) that are generalizable across biomedical research domains.
- Consider available tools and best practices for increased transparent reporting that support researchers and are generalizable across biomedical research domains.
- Discuss the roles of educational institutions, professional societies, researchers, and funders in improving computational reproducibility (*Reproducibility and Replicability in Science* Recommendation 6-6).
- Discuss how funding agencies and organizations could invest in research and development of open source, usable tools and infrastructure that support reproducibility for a broad range of studies across different domains in a seamless fashion, as well as in outreach to inform and train researchers on best practices (*Reproducibility and Replicability in Science* Recommendation 6-1).

SOURCE: Workshop agenda (available in Appendix C), September 25, 2019.

---

[1] Further information on CONSORT is available at http://www.consort-statement.org (accessed December 14, 2019).

Medical Journal Editors (ICMJE) has endorsed the CONSORT Statement and encourages journals to adopt the CONSORT guidelines for manuscripts describing clinical studies. Kiermer also mentioned the Enhancing the QUAlity and Transparency Of health Research (EQUATOR) Network, which brings together different stakeholder working groups and other collaborators and collates and promotes guidelines and resources for health research reporting.[2]

Reporting the results of studies in journals is the end of the process, after the research has already been designed and conducted, Kiermer said. She pointed out that it can be difficult for researchers to comply with reporting guidelines if they have not built the elements needed to meet those guidelines into their studies early on in the process. Improving transparency needs to begin earlier in the process, and she said that funders and institutions have a role in coordinating with journals to improve transparency in reporting.

Three panelists working in different settings shared their perspectives on lessons and best practices from clinical research that could be applied broadly across biomedical research. An-Wen Chan, Phelan Scientist at Women's College Research Institute and associate professor at the University of Toronto, described the Standard Protocol Items: Recommendations for Interventional Trials (SPIRIT) initiative as an example of how guidelines can improve the reporting of clinical trial protocols and drive quality and efficiencies downstream. Geeta Swamy, vice dean for scientific integrity and associate vice president for research at Duke University, offered her perspective on developing a culture of research integrity and accountability at an institution through education, best practices, and scientific and analytical excellence. Magali Haas, chief executive officer (CEO) and president of Cohen Veterans Bioscience, described working with strategic partners to build enabling platforms that can accelerate rigorous, reproducible, and translatable preclinical science, and discussed the various ways that funders can influence and enable reproducibility.

LESSONS FROM THE SPIRIT INITIATIVE

An-Wen Chan, Phelan Scientist, Women's College Research Institute, and Associate Professor, University of Toronto

Analyses by Chan and others have found that many clinical trial protocols lack important information on key methodological elements such

[2] Further information on the EQUATOR Network is available at https://www.equator-network.org (accessed December 14, 2019).

as primary outcomes, power calculations, or blinding, for example (see Figure 4-1). To address this, Chan and colleagues launched the SPIRIT initiative. In 2013, SPIRIT released a checklist of recommended information that should be included in a clinical trial protocol and a related paper explaining and elaborating on the supporting evidence and rationale for each item on the checklist (Chan et al., 2013a,b,c).

The SPIRIT checklist has been broadly endorsed and adopted as a standard for clinical trial protocols by more than 120 biomedical journals, Chan said. In addition, there are national ethics regulators that require submitted protocols to adhere to SPIRIT (e.g., the UK Health Research Authority), as well as funders and pharmaceutical companies that have adopted SPIRIT as the standard for their protocols. SPIRIT has been translated into six languages, and the SPIRIT website has 50,000 unique users per year.[3] Chan noted that, although most protocols are not published, more than 600 published protocols are now based on SPIRIT.

Incentives

Efforts to promote quality and transparency in research are often perceived as creating additional administrative burdens, Chan observed. To encourage adoption, efforts are being made to promote the role of SPIRIT and other guidelines in improving clinical trial efficiency.

As an example, Chan said many of the delays in Institutional Review Board (IRB) or ethics approval of clinical studies are the result of protocols

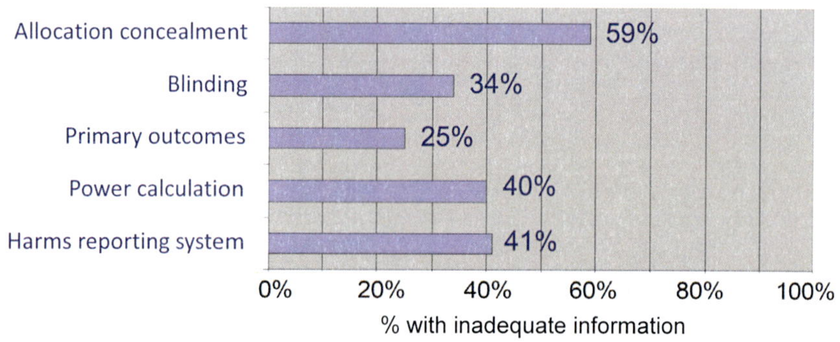

FIGURE 4-1 Important information lacking in clinical trial protocols, shown as a percentage of protocols with inadequate information.
SOURCES: Chan presentation, September 25, 2019; citing Chan et al., 2004, 2008, 2017; Hróbjartsson et al., 2009; Mhaskar et al., 2012; Pildal et al., 2005; and Scharf and Colevas, 2006.

[3] For the SPIRIT guidelines, related publications, and additional information, see https://www.spirit-statement.org (accessed November 20, 2019).

being returned for revisions due to inadequate information (Russ et al., 2009). He suggested that IRB approval time could be reduced by using the SPIRIT checklist to submit more complete protocols. Once approved, trials are often amended (three amendments per trial on average). One study of more than 3,400 industry protocols found that one third of those amendments could have been avoided if more complete information had been incorporated in the protocol at the start. The study found that each amendment delays a trial by more than 2 months, delays trial registration by about 1 month, and adds significantly to the cost of the trial (Getz et al., 2011). Adhering to reporting guidelines upfront can lead to downstream efficiencies by helping to ensure that clinical trial protocols are complete and of high quality, Chan summarized.

Enforcement

As discussed by Brian Nosek and others, rewards and incentives can inspire behavior, but enforcement is also needed. Journal editors can play a key role in adopting and enforcing policies requiring adherence to reporting guidelines or transparency initiatives, Chan said. As an example, he said clinical trial registration was proposed in the 1980s to improve transparency and quality, but was not broadly practiced until after ICMJE instituted trial registration as a requirement for publication in 2005. As noted in the first panel discussion, it is important to recognize that these policies do not come without a cost. For example, the journal *Trials* requires that every protocol submit a SPIRIT checklist. While this has increased the implementation of SPIRIT, manual checking of the protocol against the checklist is very time consuming for reviewers and editors. Simply adopting a policy is insufficient, Chan said, and enforcement requires investment of significant resources.

Funders also have enforcement power, Chan said. The National Institute for Health Research in the United Kingdom, for example, withholds a portion of a grantee's funding until a final report is published. In this way the Institute has achieved a 96 percent publication rate for their funded research (nearly twice the average rate across all types of funding agencies). Regulators have enforcement power through the implementation of legislation, although Chan noted that their authority only extends to products they regulate. IRBs can also require adherence to guidelines such as SPIRIT.

SPIRIT Electronic Protocol Tool and Resource

While the SPIRIT explanation and elaboration paper provides examples of good protocol reporting, Chan said the initiative believed it was important to build the capacity for adherence by developing a software tool and to incentivize use by providing time-saving tools. The SPIRIT Electronic Protocol Tool and Resource (SEPTRE) "aims to help investigators author their protocols more efficiently while adhering to the SPIRIT guidance," Chan said. He briefly showed participants how SEPTRE would be used to create and manage a clinical trial protocol. Drop-down menus facilitate entry of the protocol information in accordance with the SPIRIT checklist, and additional information and model examples are available. When all checklist information is entered, SEPTRE generates a formatted protocol document. SEPTRE also includes time-saving features, such as the ability to easily upload protocol information to ClinicalTrials.gov, which Chan said "reduces the registration time from hours to minutes." Another feature is the ability to automatically track protocol amendments and easily carry them through to the next protocol version.

THE INSTITUTION'S ROLE IN IMPROVING REPRODUCIBILITY

Geeta Swamy, Vice Dean for Scientific Integrity and Associate Vice President for Research, Duke University

Although it is always hoped that people know what is right and will ultimately do what is right, things can still go wrong, Swamy said, and the stakes can be high for individuals, researchers, and institutions. Regardless of whether problematic scientific research is the result of mistakes or misconduct, the consequences can include harm to research participants, loss of research funding, data loss and publication retraction, inability to recruit top faculty and students, loss of sponsor confidence, and loss of public trust, Swamy said (see Figure 4-2).

Swamy mentioned two recent cases at Duke that demonstrate the impact of research misconduct. The omics case was covered widely in scientific journals and the news media.[4] The case spanned 2006 through 2015, led to 11 retractions, and cost $10 million. Swamy said Duke runs a workshop to educate trainees and early career faculty about the omics case as many have not heard of it. The second example, a whistleblower case involving pulmonary medicine research, occurred simultaneously, but has been in the news more recently due to the time line of the investigation. This case spans 2005 to 2019 and led to 17 retractions, and the settlement cost the university $112 million.

[4] A detailed case history is presented in Appendix D of the National Academies consensus study report *Fostering Integrity in Research* (NASEM, 2017).

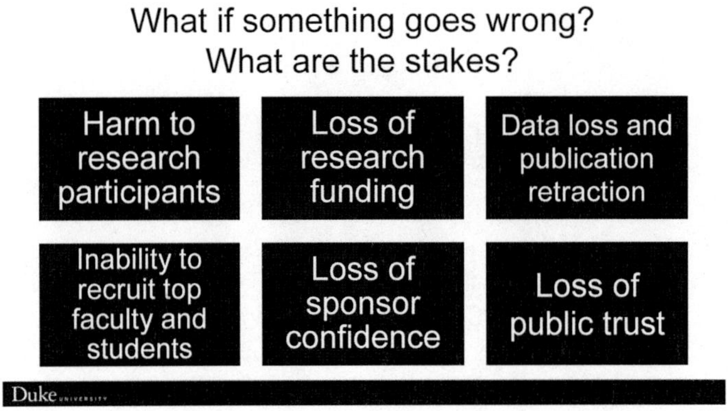

FIGURE 4-2 Some consequences of problematic scientific research.
SOURCE: Swamy presentation, September 25, 2019.

The Duke Research Integrity Culture

Swamy observed that a common theme in the workshop discussions thus far is the need for cultural change. As discussed, providing tools and resources for investigators, faculty, and trainees is important, she said, but for systematic change to occur across sectors and geographies, people must buy in to the need for change. To promote this cultural change, Duke has outlined key principles of a culture of research integrity. Swamy summarized that the research culture should be

- **Inclusive,** engaging all stakeholders in the process;
- **Comprehensive,** providing education, oversight, and accountability;
- **Multifaceted,** taking a holistic approach across all dimensions of research integrity;
- **Pragmatic,** providing the tools and resources needed to make it easier to "do the right thing"; and
- **Empowering,** enabling the research community and all stakeholders to speak up about concerns.

In its effort to support a culture of research integrity, the Duke Office of Scientific Integrity is focused on five main areas: (1) education and resources to translate the principles of integrity into routine practice; (2) standardized data management practices; (3) responsible conduct of research training for the more than 7,000 people at Duke who are engaged in research; (4) quality management strategies for both clinical and preclinical research; and (5) incident response and issue resolution. Although there are cases of misconduct, she said most incidents can be attributed to missteps, a lack of awareness, or a lack of resources.

Foundational Principles and Initiatives for Rigor, Reproducibility, and Transparency

Drawing from the work of Arturo Casadevall, Duke developed its initiatives for rigor, reproducibility, and transparency in scientific research around four foundational principles: education and training, best practice, culture and accountability, and scientific and analytical excellence (see Casadevall and Fang, 2016). Swamy described some of the initiatives in each area.

Education and Training

Education and training initiatives include responsible conduct of research (RCR) and rigor, quality, and reproducibility (RQR) training for all faculty, staff, and administrators. There are monthly town hall meetings and interactive workshops to support and promote open dialogue on integrity. Despite initial hesitation, Swamy said these are well attended and provide an opportunity for discussion of ideas and concerns. Educational resources are also provided, including an interactive board game to engage graduate students and postdoctoral fellows, and an RCR/RQR toolbox with materials for journal club-style activities that investigators can do with their laboratory members. Swamy said the intent was to empower investigators with interactive, hands-on learning resources for their trainees rather than "one more electronic module to check a box" for compliance.

Best Practice

Among the best practices implemented are electronic research notebooks for preclinical research. Swamy explained that this is a centralized, auditable system that allows for preservation and tracking of data. Data management strategies have been implemented that require all laboratories to have a data management plan, including provisions for auditing. To ensure that trainees have adequate statistical support for their analyses, they are required to use the Duke statistics core.

Culture and Accountability

As mentioned, a key principle of establishing a culture of integrity and accountability is empowering the community to be able to voice concerns, Swamy reiterated. Duke also requires every department, center, and institute to develop a science culture and accountability plan that establishes expectations of professionalism for all personnel. Compliance and oversight activities are coordinated, and there are regular communications among the units so that these activities are perceived as useful services and not as burdensome. Duke has also established a review and resolution mechanism for situations that are not already addressed by policies or regulations.

Thomas Curran asked how researchers could get more information to be able to implement the strategies discussed by Swamy at their own institutions. Swamy referred participants to a recent open-access publication describing the Duke RCR program[5] as well as her presentation from the May 2019 Research Integrity Conference.[6] She said that RCR is itself a field of research and RCR initiatives should be systematically evaluated and published so that institutions can share and implement successful strategies.

Scientific and Analytical Excellence

Swamy listed several of the Duke initiatives to promote scientific and analytical excellence. There is central review of the shared resources and core laboratories; systematic review of high-risk, high-profile investigator-initiated studies (e.g., first in human, rare disease); and external review of research programs with potential conflicts of interest (e.g., intellectual property, equity). Investigator-initiated clinical research is also subject to quality monitoring and risk-based monitoring, she said.

FUNDER/FOUNDATION ROLE IN INFLUENCING AND ENABLING REPRODUCIBILITY

Magali Haas, Chief Executive Officer and President, Cohen Veterans Bioscience

The mission of Cohen Veterans Bioscience is to accelerate the development of diagnostics and therapeutics for posttraumatic stress disorder (PTSD) and traumatic brain injury, Haas said.[7] There are few U.S. Food and Drug Administration–approved diagnostics and therapeutics for PTSD and mild traumatic brain injury. Although there are products in

---

[5] Available at https://www.tandfonline.com/doi/full/10.1080/08989621.2019.1621755 (accessed November 20, 2019).

[6] Agenda available at https://www.researchintegrity.northwestern.edu/2019conference (accessed January 13, 2020).

[7] For more information, see https://www.cohenveteransbioscience.org (accessed November 20, 2019).

the development pipeline, progress has been slow. There is much that is still not understood about the biology of these disorders, Haas said, but at the root of the slow progress are issues of reproducibility, robustness, and rigor. As a research funder, Cohen Veterans Bioscience requires quality data to make investment decisions.

Drawing on her background in pharmaceutical research and development and translational medicine, Haas recognized that the fundamental platforms and infrastructure needed to advance the field of traumatic brain injury and PTSD research were lacking. The approach of Cohen Veterans Bioscience is to work with strategic partners across industry, academia, and foundations to build those enabling platforms and foster a team science approach to accelerating product development (see Figure 4-3). "Reproducibility, robustness, and rigor are at the core of everything we do," she said.

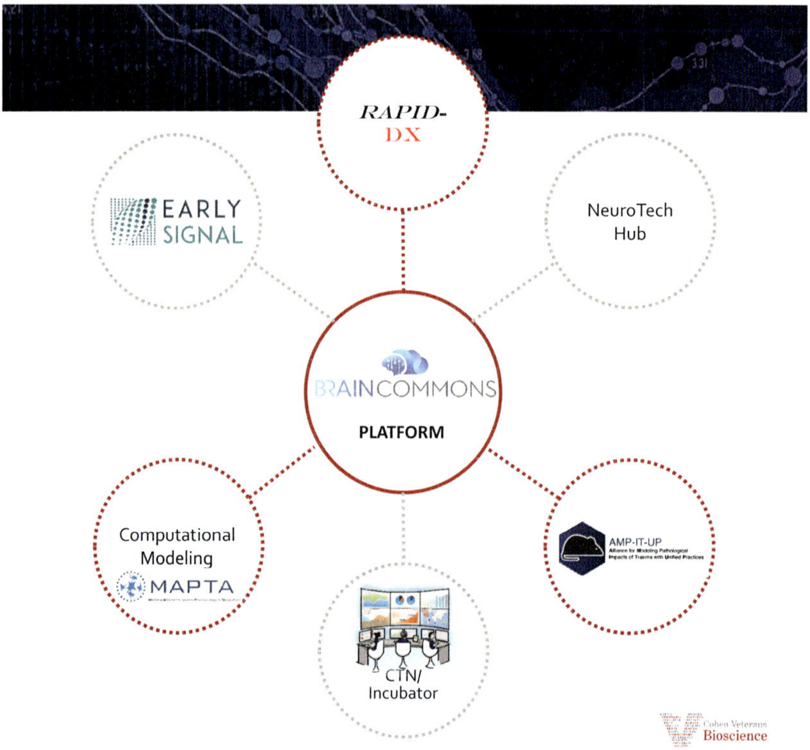

FIGURE 4-3 Cohen Veterans Bioscience platform approach to advancing reproducible, rigorous, and robust research in the field of traumatic brain injury and posttraumatic stress disorder, engaging strategic partners across industry, academia, and foundations.
SOURCE: Haas presentation, September 25, 2019.

Enabling Solutions

In 2005, Haas said, researcher John Ioannidis drew attention to the potential lack of replicability in published scientific studies (Ioannidis, 2005). Subsequent reports from industry indicated that pharmaceutical scientists were often unable to reproduce the data from studies in the literature (Prinz et al., 2011). In 2014, the National Institutes of Health (NIH) committed to taking action to enhance reproducibility (Collins and Tabak, 2014), and a range of initiatives were then launched by scientific societies, foundations, and other stakeholders. Haas described several initiatives that Cohen Veterans Bioscience has established or helped support as examples of approaches that can be adopted to influence and/or enable reproducibility.

Preclinical Data Forum

Cohen Veterans Bioscience is a grant sponsor and founding member of the Preclinical Data Forum, a network of the European College of Neuropsychopharmacology (ECNP) with more than 50 academic, industry, publishing, and research member organizations.[8] The Preclinical Data Forum focuses on enhancing reproducibility in preclinical neuroscience research. Early work sought to identify the problems and root causes, Haas said, and the focus is now on developing initiatives to address these issues.

One initiative resulting from Preclinical Data Forum efforts and described by Haas is the European Quality in Preclinical Data (EQIPD) project, which is funded by the Innovative Medicines Initiative and is focused on improving the quality of preclinical research data.[9] Another activity is the sponsorship of workshops and training programs for early career investigators on reproducibility and rigor in research. The Preclinical Data Forum has also published guidelines and checklists such as a Consensus Preclinical Checklist for information related to the use of rodents in research. Cohen Veterans Bioscience also funded a $10,000 prize, awarded through the Preclinical Data Forum, for the best negative data publication. The intent of the prize, Haas explained, is to incentivize the sharing of negative results. "The literature is extraordinarily biased toward the positive findings," she said, and as a funder investing in research, Cohen Veterans Bioscience believed it was important to incentivize a more balanced view of the data.

---

[8] Further information on the ECNP Preclinical Data Forum network is available at https://www.ecnp.eu/research-innovation/ECNP-networks/List-ECNP-Networks/Preclinical-Data-Forum (accessed December 14, 2019).

[9] Further information on the EQIPD project is available at https://quality-preclinical-data.eu (accessed December 14, 2019).

AMP-IT-UP Consortium

The AMP-IT-UP Consortium, launched by Cohen Veterans Bioscience, brings together academic and clinical researchers to address the robustness, reproducibility, and translational validity of preclinical models of brain trauma. One activity of the Consortium that Haas described is a partnership with Psychogenics, a clinical research organization (CRO), to "industrialize" animal models for PTSD and traumatic brain injury: Models developed and used in an academic setting are generally not validated for translational applications by industry, she explained, and the CRO can conduct preclinical modeling at scale. Thus far, however, efforts to reproduce some of the 16 available animal models of PTSD have been unsuccessful due to inconsistent reporting and non-standardized methods. Haas also raised the importance of funding enabling technologies that can be mass produced for use by researchers, as is being done in a consortium with the Wellcome Trust, IMEC, and the Howard Hughes Medical Institute to support a multi-channel "preclinical nanoprobe" to improve quality of the data being collected.

BRAIN Commons

Cohen Veterans Bioscience is also focused on improving data sharing and openness by sponsoring the BRAIN Commons, a cloud-based platform for data sharing of preclinical, clinical, omics, imaging, neuroimaging, and other data, Haas said. This platform, based on an open source code model, houses data in a secured environment and enables data integration and analysis across datasets and cohorts. BRAIN Commons team members are also working with NIH on incorporating preclinical common data elements. BRAIN Commons provides the infrastructure for Cohen Veterans Bioscience to require its grantees to share their results with the research community, Haas said.

Funder's Levers

In closing, Haas shared her advice regarding the levers that funders can use to influence and enable rigor, robustness, and reproducibility:

- Use the Request for Applications process as an opportunity to give feedback about the robustness of the proposed methods. Haas added that blinding grant reviewers resulted in funding decisions based on the quality of the proposal, not the investigator.
- Have intramural experts work collaboratively with the grantees and partner institutions to improve the translational potential of their research. Haas said the experts at Cohen Veterans Bioscience

have broad industry experience in areas such as data science, methodology, diagnostics development, and preclinical modeling.
- Ensure that a statistical analysis plan is developed at the outset and is executed. Haas noted that Cohen Veterans Bioscience provides statistical support for grantees because many do not have access to statistical expertise.
- Provide the tools and training needed for conducting reproducible research (e.g., the Preclinical Checklist).
- Require and provide a platform for real-time data transfer of all results (e.g., the BRAIN Commons), Haas said, and require data sharing as part of the grant agreement and enforce it by linking to milestone payments.
- Ensure sufficient funding is awarded to cover costs such as data curation and management and open publication fees.
- Invest in consortia, education, training, technologies, and platforms.

DISCUSSION

Priorities

Kiermer prompted participants to identify priorities for preclinical research. Swamy said a preproject registration process would be helpful. Haas emphasized the need for adequate funding to conduct appropriately powered experiments. There is a variety of reasons for reducing the number of animals used in a study, she said, but it is also important to remember that underpowered studies are often uninterpretable. Chan said the current practice of registration of clinical trials demonstrates the role journals can play in leading change. He suggested that journals could require preclinical protocols to be preregistered and protocols to be submitted with the manuscript reporting the final results. Journals could also develop guidance for drafting a well-defined preclinical protocol. He added that there needs to be appropriate funding and infrastructure to support researchers in meeting these requirements. Steven Goodman suggested that the highest priority for preclinical research is design. He noted that many preclinical scientists were not taught proper study design, resulting in problems from the start. He added that a survey of doctoral students found that many were taking high-level statistics analysis courses (e.g., neural networks), but had a limited statistical foundation. Chan agreed that training in study design is essential for both preclinical and clinical research, but that currently there are limited training requirements in study design for someone to conduct research studies. A participant noted the importance of recording metadata for use in data analysis. Swamy agreed and reiterated that Duke trainees are required to consult with the Duke statistics core to ensure they have the statistical capability for analysis of their data.

Protocol Development and Review

Panelists expanded on the role of IRBs in supporting transparency. Chan reiterated that IRBs can influence the design, conduct, and reporting of protocols by setting conditions such as trial registration or adherence to reporting guidelines. He noted, however, that the regulation of IRBs is highly variable across countries. In the United Kingdom, for example, research ethics committees are accountable to a national regulatory body that sets policy. In the United States, IRBs are independent and there is no central governing body. Chan observed that some IRBs require trial registration as a condition for review, and he encouraged IRBs to also recommend adherence to reporting guidelines, such as SPIRIT, to improve the content of submissions. He reiterated that is important to promote reporting guidelines to researchers as beneficial and not burdensome, in that submitting high-quality protocols facilitates more rapid review and leads to fewer queries and requests for revisions.

Swamy agreed and shared that a recent, in-depth review of the Duke Health IRB found delays were associated with the content and quality of the submissions. She suggested, however, that the primary role of an IRB is to be experts in research participant protections. IRBs are not experts in contractual publication requirements or managing conflicts of interest, nor should they be, and she raised concern about holding IRB approval "hostage" to these other interests. Duke has implemented an online tracking process for its IRB approval that allows researchers to see when each part of their submission is approved, and which sections are causing delays. The most common cause of delays is contractual agreements, she said, and she encouraged the use of standard contractual agreements, such as the Accelerated Clinical Trial Agreement that was developed by a group of Clinical and Translational Science Awards (CTSA) program investigators.[10]

Chan agreed that IRBs are overburdened and underresourced, and suggested that a separate institutional arm could take on the review of protocols for quality and transparency elements. He noted that some investigators question why the quality of the science in their submissions is being examined in an ethics review. Chan said quality and ethics are closely related, and a poorly designed study can be unethical.

Swamy pointed out that the investigator is not necessarily the author of the protocol. In industry, for example, the protocol might be written

[10] For model agreements, see https://www.ara4us.org (accessed November 20, 2019).

by someone with specialized expertise in the regulatory requirements, working in collaboration with the investigators. She said protocols written with the assistance of a regulatory coordinator tend to progress more quickly through IRB review than an early career investigator-initiated and -written protocol. Haas agreed and added that many early career faculty have no background or experience in topics such as informed consent.

Chan described a study comparing the information in IRB-approved clinical trial protocols to information for the same trials in the clinical trial registry. For more than one-fifth of the studies evaluated, the primary outcomes in the protocol did not match those entered in the trial registry. He suggested that concordance of this information should be checked prospectively or made public so that those interested could conduct their own assessments. In addition, he said that using an electronic tool as the database for protocol information, such as SEPTRE, could help to ensure that information is consistent because protocol information can be exported from the tool to the IRB and the trial registry.

Haas raised the possibility of linking final publications back to the original protocol. Chan referred to the work of Altman on the concept of threaded publications, linking all publications that stem from a given protocol/registered clinical trial. Chan and Swamy mentioned the concept of a common identifier or "universal object identifier" for protocols that could be preserved across the different platforms used by journals, IRBs, and others.

Goodman asked how protocol review could be made a routine part of funding decisions, and how adherence to proposed protocols might be monitored after grants are awarded. Swamy noted that there are new requirements for the Human Subjects and Clinical Trials Information Form to be submitted to NIH with proposal and grant applications. Although a full protocol is not required, she said that a synopsis, primary outcome, and eligibility criteria must be included. She did not know the extent to which adherence to the proposed plans would continue to be evaluated over the course of the grant, but suggested that this information could be part of the annual progress report. Swamy noted that the recent update to the Common Rule removed the requirement to determine concordance between the grant and the protocol. This was done, in part, because protocols can change between when the grant application is submitted and when IRB approval is received. She suggested there is a need to find other ways to ensure consistency.

Funding for Development and Sustainability

Leslie McIntosh, co-founder and CEO of Ripeta, asked about securing funding to implement automated solutions. Chan said the development of the SEPTRE tool was funded by interested government entities, including the Canadian Institutes of Health Research, the National Cancer Institute of Canada, and the Canadian Agency for Drugs and Technologies in Health. He noted that securing grants for the development of tools is challenging because these types of projects are not answering a research question. Once developed, it is difficult to fund the maintenance of the tools. One approach under consideration is a subscription model, Chan said, adding that researchers from lower income countries could access the tool for free. He noted that one potential source of support is investment by institutions that recognize the importance of promoting transparency and improving completeness of protocols.

Swamy said Duke leverages CTSA funds for new initiatives, but noted that CTSA funds are for developing solutions, not maintaining them once they are operational. Once a new initiative is operational, she said, a business proposal is presented to the leadership of the school of medicine and the university. All programs are assessed for impact, effectiveness, and acceptability, and that information is used to support the case for internal funding to support these programs.

Investigating Misconduct

Yvette Carter, health scientist administrator in the Office of Research Integrity (ORI) at NIH, said that like the journals, ORI does not conduct investigations. They are conducted by the awardee's institution. She suggested that instead of contacting authors with concerns of misconduct, journal editors could contact the research integrity officer at the author's institutions, or ORI at NIH, as appropriate. She urged contact "earlier rather than later." She added that ORI can provide image analysis expertise to assist in investigations. Carter asked Swamy what lessons from the recent misconduct investigations at Duke could the ORI Division of Education and Integrity share to improve research integrity. The most recent case involved the "overwhelming fabrication of data," Swamy said. While it is always exciting for investigators to get good results, she emphasized the importance of looking at raw data, test results, and data outputs, not just the final tables or figures or summary data for inclusion in a manuscript, to confirm that the findings make sense.

Common Data Elements

Stuart Hoffman, scientific program manager for the Department of Veterans Affairs' Office of Research and Development, shared his experience with the development of common data elements for traumatic brain injury and noted the challenges of coming to consensus on those elements. As common data elements are now being considered for preclinical research, he raised the issue of novel methods that do not conform to common data elements, and the possibility that research could be steered toward techniques for which common data elements do exist.

Haas said common data elements are essential to enable the sharing and analysis of data across systems. Data platforms, such as the BRAIN Commons, rely on common data elements and standards, she said. She agreed that development of common data elements for preclinical research will be challenging, and noted that NIH has assembled a preclinical common data elements working group. The extent to which the common data elements are adopted depends on incentives and enforcement ("carrots and sticks"). She noted the need to educate the research community on the benefits of using common data elements for reproducibility and independent validation of studies.

5

Checklists and Guidelines

Highlights of Key Points Made by Individual Speakers

- Checklists can improve transparent reporting and impact research practice, but endorsement by journals is insufficient. Checklists should be mandatory and compliance must be monitored even though this approach adds burden on authors, and is resource intensive for journals to implement. (Macleod, Swaminathan)
- Not all checklist items are relevant for all conditions, and there is often a lack of agreement by checklist assessors when evaluating compliance of a manuscript. (Macleod)
- Checklist items should be prioritized and pilot tested to determine whether they are meaningful for the end users. (Goodman, Silberberg)
- Although transparent reporting occurs at the end of the research process, there is a need to improve the rigor of research from the start. (Coller, Swaminathan)
- Few institutions provide formal training in the design and conduct of research. Developing a free, comprehensive, modular, adaptable, and upgradable educational resource would eliminate the need for institutions to invest time and resources in creating their own. (Silberberg)

- Grassroots initiatives and communities of champions are needed to support culture change by all stakeholders. (Coller, Silberberg)
- Evaluating research quality initiatives is important to show that an intervention is achieving the intended outcome. (Macleod)

Among the best practices discussed during the second panel session were guidelines and checklists (see Chapter 4). In this session, panelists delved further into the practical application and effectiveness of guidelines and checklists for enhancing transparent reporting of biomedical research (see Box 5-1 for corresponding workshop session objectives).

Sowmya Swaminathan, head of editorial policy and research integrity at Nature Research, and Malcolm Macleod discussed the impacts of several current checklists and provided an overview of the Minimum Standards Working Group's development and pilot testing of the materials, design, analysis, and reporting (MDAR) framework and checklist. Shai Silberberg discussed the uptake and effectiveness of checklists and strategies for improving adherence. The session was moderated by Barry

BOX 5-1
Workshop Session Objectives

- Discuss journal and funder assessments of researchers' adherence to transparent reporting guidelines, including discussion of the effectiveness of checklists.
  - Highlight empirical assessments of checklist application from funders, journals, and researchers; and
  - Consider practical application and effectiveness of checklists and guidelines to encourage or require transparent reporting of preclinical biomedical research.
- Discuss how funders could require thoughtful discussion in grant applications of how uncertainties will be evaluated, along with any relevant issues regarding replicability and computational reproducibility (*Reproducibility and Replicability in Science* Recommendation 6-9).
- Discuss how journals and scientific societies could disclose their policies relevant to achieving reproducibility and replicability, and how journals could be encouraged to set and implement desired standards of reproducibility and replicability and adopt policies to reduce the likelihood of non-replicability (*Reproducibility and Replicability in Science* Recommendation 6-7).

SOURCE: Workshop agenda (available in Appendix C), September 25, 2019.

Coller, physician in chief, vice president for medical affairs, and David Rockefeller Professor at The Rockefeller University.

To open the panel session, Coller described an early example of the successful use of a checklist from *The Checklist Manifesto* by Atul Gawande (2009). In 1935, the U.S. Army held a competition to award a contract for production of a new long-range bomber. Boeing's entry, the Model 299 (later designated the B-17), was superior to the other entries in key areas such as design, payload capacity, and performance. However, during an evaluation flight, the anticipated winner of the contract climbed, stalled, and crashed, killing the pilot and a crewmember. The investigation concluded that the crash was the result of "pilot error due to an unprecedented complexity" of the plane, Coller said. The experienced pilot had failed to release the lock on the elevator and rudder controls, and it was said at the time that the Model 299 was "too much plane for one man to fly," Coller relayed. Boeing lost the contract and came close to bankruptcy.

Still interested in the technology, the Army purchased several Model 299s and worked with test pilots to improve safety. As the original test pilot was highly trained, it was concluded that additional training was not the answer. The solution they reached, Coller said, was to create a concise, step-by-step checklist for takeoff, landing, and taxiing that would fit on an index card. Ultimately, nearly 13,000 B-17 bombers were built, and pilots logged 1.8 million miles without any further accidents.

Coller listed several of the lessons learned about flying a B-17 safely in 1935 and adapted them to a performing and reporting science in 2019. First, he said the alignment of incentives for flying the plane safely are absolute because not flying safely can result in death. For performing and reporting science, the alignment of incentives is "more nuanced and subtle." Coller described the complexity of flying a plane safely in 1935 as analogue (e.g., dials, binary switches), while science today exists in the digital world. Although pilots needed to make many decisions to fly the B-17 safely, the number of decisions was finite; however, he said the number of decisions involved in performing and reporting science today is "virtually infinite." A B-17 pilot's dependence on others involved a limited team, while performing and reporting science depends on a greatly expanded universe of others. Finally, Coller said, the dependence on "black boxes" by pilots in 1935 was finite and he noted they could actually "kick the tires." In science, what happens in the black boxes can be vital, and it is increasingly difficult to know the quality (e.g., an error in one line of code in one algorithm can have far-reaching effects if that algorithm is used widely).[1]

---

[1] A black box in the context of the sciences refers to part of a process or pathway between the inputs and the outputs for which the mechanisms are unknown or are not well understood by the user.

CHECKLIST IMPLEMENTATION BY LIFE SCIENCE JOURNALS: TOWARD MINIMUM REPORTING STANDARDS FOR RESEARCH

Sowmya Swaminathan, Head, Editorial Policy and Research Integrity, Nature Research
Malcolm Macleod, Professor of Neurology and Translational Neuroscience, University of Edinburgh

Swaminathan and Macleod described several examples of checklist initiatives leading up to the creation of the Minimum Standards Working Group, a group of journal editors and experts on reproducibility that has developed minimum standards for reporting in life sciences.[2]

As background, Macleod shared an example of how poor preclinical study quality can lead to bias in published animal studies, resulting in serious implications for translation to clinical trials. The neuroprotective drug, NXY-059, was shown to be efficacious in animal studies, but the drug was ineffective in a large clinical trial. A systematic review of the published animal studies revealed that, although the overall animal data supported the efficacy conclusion, the majority of the studies did not report randomization, blinded conduct of the experiment, and blinded outcome assessment. The few studies that were of high quality (randomized and blinded) reported significantly lower treatment efficacy (Macleod et al., 2008).

To understand the scale of the problem, Macleod and colleagues assessed the publications included in the Research Assessment Exercise, which evaluated the quality of research at five leading UK institutions. More than 1,000 publications involving animal research were assessed for their reporting of the four key items recommended by Landis and colleagues as the minimum necessary for transparent reporting: blinding, inclusion and exclusion criteria, randomization, and sample size calculation (Landis et al., 2012). Macleod found that less than 20 percent reported blinding, 10 percent reported inclusion and exclusion criteria, 15 percent of the papers reported randomization, and 2 percent reported power calculations. Overall, he said, 68 percent of the papers assessed reported none of these elements, and one paper reported doing all of them. These types of examples have led to a range of initiatives to improve research, including various guidelines and checklists.

---

[2] The formation of the working group is described here: https://osf.io/preprints/metaarxiv/9sm4x (accessed December 14, 2019).

Checklists as a Solution

Nature *Journals Reporting Checklist for Life Science Papers*

In 2013, Nature Research announced the implementation of measures to improve the reporting of life science research published in its journals.[3] A key component of this initiative, Swaminathan said, was the development of a reporting checklist that authors are now required to include with their manuscript submission.[4] The checklist helps to facilitate more complete reporting of study details, establishes expectations for reporting of statistics, and provides journal policies on the sharing of data and code. The author's completed checklist is provided to the peer reviewers and journal editors who monitor compliance.

A 2017 survey of authors who had published in *Nature* journals found that 83 percent of respondents said "the checklist had significantly improved reporting of statistics within papers published in *Nature* journals," Swaminathan said. Respondents also perceived improved reporting of reagents and animal models, and increased data deposition in public repositories (see Figure 5-1, panel A). Although the primary goal of implementing the checklist was to improve reporting quality in published papers, Swaminathan said that it was hoped that it might also raise awareness and impact research practice. In this regard, 78 percent of respondents said they continue to use the checklist to some extent in their own work, regardless of planned journal submission (see Figure 5-1, panel B).[5]

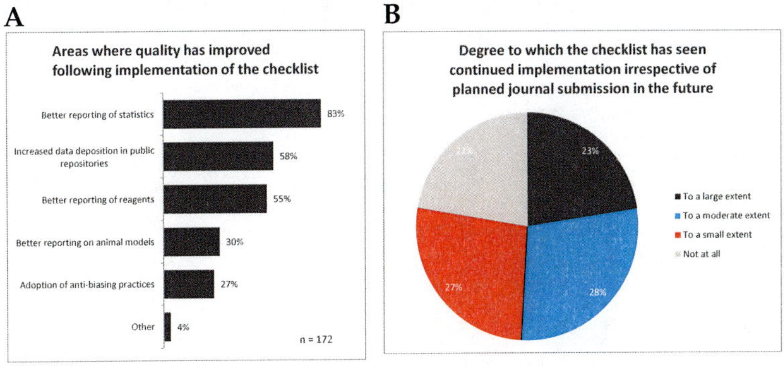

FIGURE 5-1 Impact of checklist on published papers and research practice.
SOURCES: Swaminathan presentation, September 25, 2019, from the 2017 survey of published *Nature* journal authors (Nature Research, 2018, and footnote 5 below).

---

[3] See https://www.nature.com/news/polopoly_fs/1.12852!/menu/main/topColumns/topLeftColumn/pdf/496398a.pdf (accessed November 20, 2019).

[4] Available at https://media.nature.com/full/nature-assets/ncomms/authors/ncomms_lifesciences_checklist.pdf (accessed November 20, 2019).

[5] For complete data and related materials, see https://figshare.com/articles/Nature_Reproducibility_survey_2017/6139937 (accessed November 20, 2019).

Summarizing the experience with the Nature Research journals checklist, Swaminathan said the use of checklists can improve reporting standards and impact research practice, but she emphasized that checklists need to be mandatory and compliance must be monitored. She acknowledged that mandates pose additional burdens for authors, and monitoring compliance is resource intensive. In addition, researchers must contend with a wide diversity of policies from their institutions, funders, and publishers. Journals are "at the end of the process," she said, and achieving a broad shift in research practice will require initiatives targeting the beginning, within laboratories and academic institutions.

Nature Publishing Group Quality in Publication (NPQIP) Study

Another study, described by Macleod, assessed the impact of the Nature Research reporting checklist for life science papers. The study evaluated reporting quality in published papers that had been submitted after the policy requiring checklist completion was implemented by *Nature*, compared with reporting quality in publications that had been submitted to *Nature* journals before policy implementation, and also to similar papers published in other (non-*Nature*) journals. Macleod reported that there were substantial increases in reporting of all four of the items identified by Landis (blinding, reporting inclusions and exclusions, randomization, and sample size calculation) after the requirement for checklist submission was implemented by Nature Publishing Group (NPQIP Collaborative Group, 2019). NPQIP demonstrates that "a checklist, on its own, is not enough," Macleod said.

Minimum Standards Working Group

The Minimum Standards Working Group includes editors and experts in reproducibility from Nature Research, the Public Library of Science, Science/American Association for the Advancement of Science, Cell Press, eLIFE, Wiley, the Center for Open Science, and the University of Edinburgh. The aim of the working group was to "improve transparency and reproducibility by defining minimum reporting standards in life sciences," which Swaminathan said includes biological, biomedical, and preclinical research. She added that the working group, assembled in 2017, was inspired by the success of the International Committee of Medical Journal Editors in influencing clinical trial reporting and the impact of the Consolidated Standards of Reporting Trials (CONSORT) checklist.

The working group consulted with external experts and stakeholders and referenced existing journal checklists and policy frameworks (including the Nature Research checklist, Enhancing the QUAlity and Transparency Of health Research [EQUATOR] Network guidelines, and Transparency and Openness Promotion [TOP] guidelines mentioned in

Appendix B, and others). The work was also informed by meta-research on the implementation of checklists and the National Academies consensus study reports *Reproducibility and Replicability in Science* (NASEM, 2019) and *Open Science by Design* (NASEM, 2018).

The working group issued the following three key outputs:

- A **minimum standards framework,** which establishes minimum expectations of transparency across the core areas of materials, design, analysis, and reporting;
- A **minimum standards checklist,** which is an implementation tool to facilitate compliance with the framework; and
- An **elaboration document,** which provides context for the minimum standards framework and guidance for using the checklist.

The three documents have been publicly released as the MDAR Framework, the MDAR Checklist for Authors, and the MDAR Framework and Checklist Elaboration Document, and Swaminathan encouraged participants to provide feedback.[6] The target audiences for the deliverables are journals and publishing platforms, as well as research institutions, funders, and other stakeholders, she said. The framework and checklist are broadly applicable across the research life cycle, from study design and grant submission through to manuscript submission, peer review, and publication, and are also intended as a teaching tool.

MDAR Framework Elements

Swaminathan elaborated on the four reporting categories of the MDAR framework, listing the key elements that the working group identified for each:

- "**Materials:** biological reagents, lab animals, model organisms, animals in the field, unique specimens
- **Design:** study/experimental design, protocols, statistics, methodologies, dual-use research consent
- **Analysis:** data, code, statistics as relevant to analysis
- **Reporting:** discipline-specific guidelines and standards."

The framework also discusses two levels of reporting, the "minimum" required level and a recommended "best practice" level, both of

---

[6] The three key outputs of the Minimum Standards Working Group are available at https://osf.io/xfpn4 (accessed November 20, 2019), https://osf.io/bj3mu (accessed November 20, 2019), and https://osf.io/xzy4s (accessed November 20, 2019), respectively.

which include information on the accessibility and unambiguous identification of the elements reported. By adopting the MDAR framework, Swaminathan said, a stakeholder is committing to incorporate the minimum standards into their policies.

MDAR Checklist Pilot Testing

Author and Editor Perceptions Survey

The first objectives of the MDAR pilot test were to collect authors' and editors' perceptions of the checklist (e.g., usefulness, accessibility, missing elements, impact on manuscript processing times). Surveys were done of editors from 13 journals,[7] and of 211 authors completing checklists (see Figure 5-2). Swaminathan summarized that the majority of authors found the checklist tool to be helpful, with 44 percent of authors responding "very helpful" and 36 percent responding "somewhat helpful."[8] The

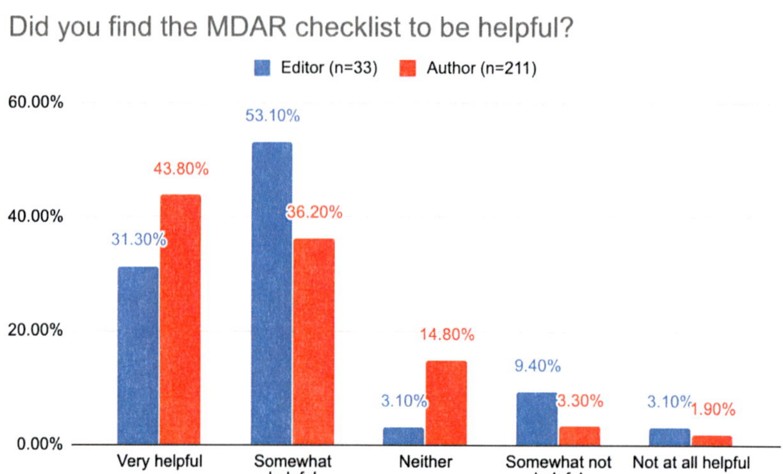

FIGURE 5-2 Editor and author experiences with the MDAR checklist.
NOTE: MDAR = materials, design, analysis, and reporting.
SOURCES: Swaminathan presentation, September 25, 2019. This figure is taken from the presentation, "Summary results of author and editor responses. MDAR working group, September 2019," available at https://osf.io/znq64 (accessed December 14, 2019).

---

[7] *BMC Microbiology, Ecology & Evolution, eLife, EMBO journals, Epigenetics, F1000R, Molecular Cancer Therapeutics, Microbiology Open, PeerJ, PLOS Biology, PNAS, Science, Scientific Reports.*

[8] Complete data from the author and editor surveys are available at https://osf.io/gqsmp (accessed November 20, 2019).

majority of editors also found the MDAR checklist helpful, with 31 percent of editors responding "very helpful" and 53 percent responding "somewhat helpful."

Evaluation of the MDAR Checklist Experience

Macleod described another evaluation of 289 manuscripts submitted to the same 13 journals. On average, editors spent 24 minutes assessing checklist performance. Only 15 of the 42 items on the checklist were relevant for more than 50 percent of the manuscripts. Macleod noted that this is not unexpected for an overarching guideline. For example, he said, a checklist item about plant-based research would not be relevant to studies that do not involve plants. Editors assessed the relevance of checklist items in the areas of materials, design, analysis, and reporting, and the extent to which they believed authors had complied. Macleod observed that there were many areas where assessors believed an item was highly relevant, but determined that few authors were reporting those items, and vice versa, where items were deemed to be irrelevant, but were highly reported.

Eighty-nine of the manuscripts were dual-evaluated by two independent assessors and agreement was determined using Kappa statistics (which Macleod explained subtracts chance agreement). Assessors agreed on the relevance of some checklist items, but for others "the agreement was not much better than [it] is by chance alone," Macleod said. Similarly, for checklist items that both assessors agreed were relevant, there was not necessarily agreement on whether the manuscript had met the guideline criteria for reporting of the item. He noted that the confidence intervals for the Kappa scores were wide.

MDAR Experience Summary and Next Steps

Macleod summarized that "authors and editors seem to like the checklist and find it useful," and "the time taken to check performance is short." He suggested that spending more time per checklist item might have resulted in greater agreement among the dual assessors. Not all checklist items are relevant at all times, and a "dynamic checklist" that offers fields relevant for a particular journal, for example, might be useful. Agreement between assessors was limited, and confidence intervals were wide, but the areas of disagreement should be highlighted as areas to focus on with regard to clarity of the checklist item and the information provided in the elaboration and explanation document.

The next steps in the development of the MDAR checklist, Macleod and Swaminathan said, will be a consultation with key stakeholders and interested individuals, and revisions of the checklist and supporting materials per the feedback.

APPROACHES TO IMPROVE ADHERENCE TO CHECKLISTS AND GUIDELINES[9]

Shai Silberberg, Director of Research Quality, National Institute of Neurological Disorders and Stroke

By definition, Silberberg said, a guideline is "a general rule, principle, or piece of advice." In other words, a guideline is a suggestion to be taken into consideration for the longer term, he said, and guidelines are not generally effective at changing behavior. A checklist, by definition, is "a list of items required, things to be done, or points to be considered, used as a reminder." Checklists are for the specific task at hand, he said.

Less Is More

A systematic review published in 2012 compared the completeness of reporting of randomized controlled trials in journals that had endorsed CONSORT versus those that had not (Turner et al., 2012). The most significant difference found was for the checklist item allocation concealment, which was reported adequately in 45 percent of the trials in the journals that endorsed CONSORT versus 22 percent of the trials in non-endorsing journals. While twice the reporting rate is impressive improvement, Silberberg pointed out that more than 50 percent of the trials published in the CONSORT-endorsing journals did not follow the guidelines. He suggested that the length of the checklist is a contributing factor to this noncompliance. Allocation concealment is very important for reducing selection bias, but it is just one of 38 items on the 2010 CONSORT. When faced with a long checklist, Silberberg said, important items can be overlooked.

"Less can be more," Silberberg said, and he discussed the need to stage priorities. The CONSORT checklist was implemented more than two decades ago, and yet complete reporting of trial information is still lacking. He suggested a more concise checklist, "a minimum set of items that are the most crucial not to ignore." After researchers are trained in the highest priority elements and have adopted the desired behaviors, they should then implement the next set of priority items, and so forth, continuing to stage introduction over the longer term, he suggested.

[9] Silberberg stated that the opinions expressed in his presentations are his own and are not official opinions of the National Institutes of Health.

As recommended by Landis and colleagues, "At a minimum, studies should report on sample size estimation, whether and how animals were randomized, whether investigators were blind to the treatment, and the handling of data" (Landis et al., 2012, p. 187). Silberberg said there is a high risk of bias associated with these items and they form the foundation of a rigorous study. He emphasized that if the data are of poor quality, then all that follows (analysis, reporting) is of little value.

Shared Responsibility for Cultural Change

Silberberg noted that the Landis publication on transparent reporting was an output of a 2012 National Institute of Neurological Disorders and Stroke (NINDS) stakeholder workshop in improving the design and reporting of animal studies (Landis et al., 2012). Another conclusion of the 2012 NINDS workshop, he said, was that all stakeholders share responsibility. He observed that the discussions at this National Academies workshop have also emphasized the roles of all stakeholders, and he encouraged participants to ask themselves what they can contribute to creating change and promoting transparent reporting.

The need for change in the research culture has been raised throughout this National Academies workshop, Silberberg said, and changing the culture requires education and a change to the incentive structure. NINDS convened a workshop in 2018 to evaluate the extent to which scientists receive formal training in the design and conduct of research.[10] A survey of 41 institutions with NINDS-funded training grants found that only 5 offered a full-length course on the principles of rigorous research, and Silberberg said that all of the elements of rigorous research cannot be covered in one course. Other institutions provided lectures (17) or minicourses (2), but 12 provided no formal training (and 5 did not respond to the survey).

In considering why so few institutions provide formal training in research principles, Silberberg suggested that building an educational program "from scratch" is difficult and requires a significant investment of time, knowledge and expertise, motivation, and funding. He proposed the development of a free educational resource that institutions could use for their own training programs, eliminating the need to invest energy and resources in creating their own. The resource would be comprehensive, modular, adaptable, and upgradable.

---

[10] See https://www.ninds.nih.gov/News-Events/Events-Proceedings/Events/Visionary-Resource-Instilling-Fundamental-Principles-Rigorous (accessed November 20, 2019).

Creating Communities of Champions

Silberberg summarized the recommendations from the 2018 NINDS workshop. First, "an effective educational platform should target all career stages." Silberberg noted that the first panel of this National Academies workshop emphasized the importance of targeting trainees and early career scientists in particular. He added that many senior investigators also need training on the principles of rigorous research. Next, a culture change is needed at all levels of academic, publishing, and funding organizations. This includes a change to the incentive structure. Third, "academic institutions need to play a proactive role in changing the culture," Silberberg said. He noted that institutions are often missing from the discussions of research culture, and tenure, promotion, and hiring committees within institutions play a central role in the research culture.

Attendees at the 2018 NINDS workshop suggested that to achieve these goals, a "grassroots effort" is needed, Silberberg said. They called for "the establishment of communities of champions within and across institutions to share resources, change culture, and support better training at all academic levels."

Each stakeholder organization has champions for culture change, Silberberg said. To bring them together, NINDS has created a mechanism on its website for champions of rigorous research practices to self-identify and connect with others in their institution.[11] NINDS is currently considering how best to support interactions of these communities of champions with others regionally, nationally, and even globally.

In closing, Silberberg shared an example of how communities of champions can foster improved transparency of presentations at scientific meetings (Silberberg et al., 2017). A short conference talk or poster does not generally allow for sufficient depth of information for attendees to have a sense of the rigor of the work. One approach to increasing transparency, Silberberg said, is to provide more detail in figures (e.g., individual data points, total number of samples). Another approach, he said, is to add symbols or "rigor emojis" to the figures to indicate that the study was, for example, randomized, blinded, or confirmatory (see Figure 5-3).

---

[11] See https://www.ninds.nih.gov/Current-Research/Trans-Agency-Activities/Rigor-Transparency/RigorChampionsAndResources (accessed November 20, 2019).

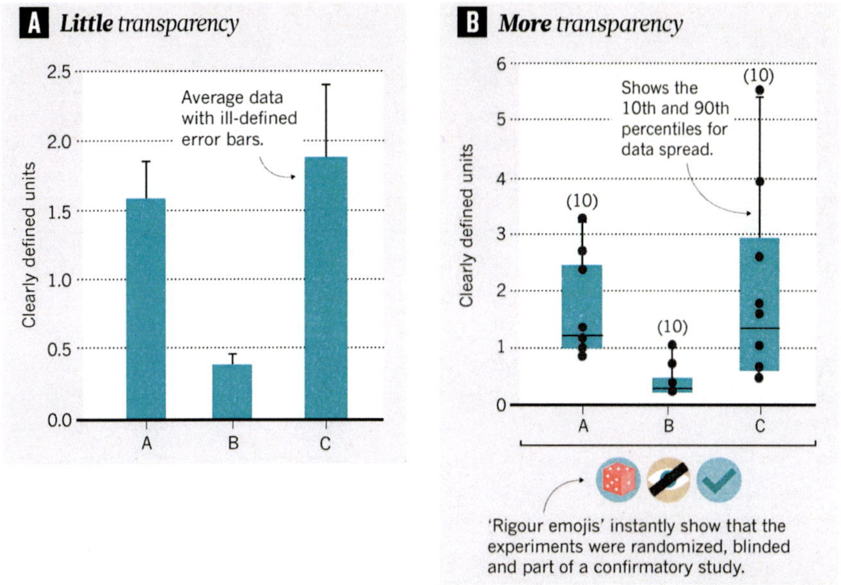

FIGURE 5-3 Proposed strategy to improve transparent reporting in conference posters.
SOURCES: Silberberg presentation, September 24, 2019; Silberberg et al., 2017.

DISCUSSION

Motivating Action: Champions for Culture Change

During the discussion, panelists expanded on the topic of the need for champions of culture change, including the need for grassroots efforts and what motivates stakeholders to take action.

Institutional Leadership

Coller observed that, although the focus of the workshop is transparent reporting, it has been noted throughout the discussions that reporting is the end of the process, and there should be more attention to improving the rigor of research from the start. He asked panelists what institutional leaders should be doing to promote rigorous science. He supported the concept of a community of champions, as discussed by Silberberg, and proposed the creation of a "research integrity advocate" that would be comparable to the research participant advocate position established at NIH-funded clinical research centers. The research integrity advocate could be the institutional champion tasked with promoting culture change, he said.

Macleod noted that many of the institutions that have established practices to promote a rigorous research culture have been highly motivated by the need to address an incident of research malpractice. He suggested that focusing efforts primarily on addressing misconduct and preventing falsification, fabrication, and plagiarism is the wrong approach, and institutions should instead emphasize improving research performance broadly for the benefit of all.

Silberberg countered the comment that reporting is the end of the process. Science is a continuous cycle he said, and journals might be at the end of one round, but they are the beginning of the next round in that publications are then used to justify the next grant proposal or the next research plan. He agreed that journals are not responsible for enforcing rigorous science, but they have a role to play in increasing transparency. As an example, he mentioned the checklist required by *Nature* journals that allows peer reviewers to better assess the rigor of the study being reported. He suggested that major stakeholders are often hesitant to be the first to take action because of the potential financial ramifications. For example, university leadership will continue to push investigators to publish frequently in high-profile journals, potentially at the expense of rigor, because that is what is valued and rewarded by grant reviewers. He reiterated the need for champions and grassroots initiatives to push for change by all the major stakeholders.

Grassroots Stakeholder Efforts

As an example of a grassroots approach to championing rigorous science, Macleod mentioned the UK Reproducibility Network. The network includes self-organized local groups of early career researchers who connect for mentoring and journal clubs that promote openness and reproducibility; stakeholders (e.g., journals, funders); and academic institutions. Macleod added that academic institutions seeking to join must formally commit to promoting rigorous research and must appoint an Academic Lead for Research Improvement that is a senior-level position. Joining the UK Reproducibility Network, he said, provides a mechanism for local communities of early career researchers and their institutions to commit to creating an improved research culture without waiting to be motivated by a public misconduct scandal.

Kelly Dunham, senior manager for strategic initiatives at the Patient-Centered Outcomes Research Institute (PCORI), described the Ensuring Value in Research Funders' Forum as an example of a grassroots stakeholder effort.[12] The forum, established in 2016, includes about 40 funding organizations and has issued a consensus statement and guiding principles intended to maximize the probability of impact of the research funded, she explained. The forum is working to "characterize what good practice looks like," she said, and to develop minimum standards and recommendations for the larger biomedical research ecosystem. She said there is occasional pushback from some funders that a particular approach is not practicable, and she emphasized the importance of sharing examples of successes learning from each other. Dunham said funders can play a role in ensuring the results of the studies they fund are made publicly available, and PCORI has taken on the responsibility of providing transparent and well-documented results to the public. PCORI has a process of peer review for all of its funded research and publicly releases lay summaries and clinical summaries of studies.

Cindy Sheffield, project manager of the Alzheimer's Disease Preclinical Efficacy Database (AlzPED) for NIH, referred participants to AlzPED, which she said currently includes about 900 articles "that have been evaluated for 24 elements of experimental design."[13] A goal of AlzPED is to create awareness and work toward changing the culture. She said that although they cannot evaluate rigor and transparency quantitatively, they do check and record in the database whether the elements of design are reported or not.

The Role of the Investigator

Swaminathan observed that stakeholders are increasingly aware of the problem of irreproducibility and seem interested in taking action. She noted that a survey of researchers found that they believe researchers are responsible for addressing issues of reproducibility, but a supportive institutional infrastructure (e.g., training, mentoring, funding, publishing) is needed.

Silberberg said a senior scientist can have difficulty accepting that the work they have done over the past several decades might not have been of the highest quality. Coller added that having buy-in from senior investigators is essential to effect culture change, and senior investigators are needed as champions as well. Training grants are important, he said, but institutional culture is not defined by trainees and early career investigators. Arturo Casadevall called on the scientific elite to step up and require rigorous research. "Most scientists today want to do rigorous good sci-

[12] See https://sites.google.com/view/evir-funders-forum/home (accessed November 20, 2019).

[13] See https://alzped.nia.nih.gov (accessed November 20, 2019).

ence, and the problem is they are caught in a system in which they are not judged by it," he said. As discussed, much of the effort to change the culture of research has been from editors and grassroots efforts, he said, and few leading scientists have taken a stand on this issue. He lamented that the most respected scientific leaders "are often the most silent," and are hesitant to criticize the system through which they have come up.

Cross-Sector Coordination

John Gardinier agreed with the emphasis on changing the research culture and noted in particular the need to address the impact of silos in research, including the potential for conflicting information being published by different scientific disciplines. Macleod said he had experience with different disease research communities each asserting that the others had issues with research rigor, but they did not. He said he encourages them to do a systematic review of the quality of reporting in their field, and many come to the conclusion that they do, in fact, have a problem.

Checklists and Study Design

Swaminathan said there is still a lack of general consensus regarding what is a "good study." She said she and others believe the four items recommended by Landis and colleagues "not only should be reported, but should be incorporated into study design." Most studies, however, do not incorporate these elements, and if these elements are reported in a publication, it is generally due to an enforcement and compliance mechanism. Coller agreed and observed that there is often agreement on what constitutes "bad science" and perhaps driving consensus on what is bad research form is a place to start.

Veronique Kiermer said that the ultimate goal is conducting well-designed studies, and that addressing study design through the implementation of a reporting checklist is a "very convoluted" approach. However, she was impressed by Swaminathan's data that showed researchers were continuing to use the reporting checklists in their ongoing work, suggesting that checklists do have an educational aspect. Macleod said institutions can assess how their research measures up against a checklist, then work to improve in areas that are deficient, and reward the investigators who contribute to that improvement with promotion and tenure. Steven Goodman said the checklists discussed are not user friendly. He supported the concept of prioritizing key items and proposed pilot testing checklists to determine what might be useful for end users.

Another problem, as illustrated by dual evaluation of the MDAR checklist discussed by Macleod, is the lack of agreement by checklist assessors on the compliance of a manuscript. Swaminathan emphasized the need for better coordination of concepts and language across the different stakeholders and different stages of the research process. She noted that a goal of the Minimal Standards Working Group was to establish a minimum standard that would be applicable across the research life cycle. Macleod noted that there have been efforts to coordinate the language between MDAR and the Animal Research: Reporting of In Vivo Experiments (ARRIVE) guidelines so that relevant sections are interoperable, and that tools are in development to automate assessment of checklists. He added that disagreement among assessors and peer reviewers on whether a paper meets a particular standard is often related more to the assessor's lack of understanding of the concepts (e.g., the unit of assessment, biological versus technical replicates) than the language used in the checklist instrument. Swaminathan agreed and said in implementing the Nature Research checklist, for example, they found that authors conflated the experimental unit with the number of times an experiment had been replicated, presented aggregate data from multiple experiments as if from a single experiment, and confused technical and biological replicates. The extent to which this occurred varied by field, more so in fields "that are inherently qualitative and descriptive, but that as science has evolved, have been forced into a quantitative mold."

Assessment and Accountability

Yarimar Carrasquillo observed that the discussions have focused on training for students and early career investigators and on checklists for reporting studies, and suggested that institutions and funding agencies need to also implement checkpoints between those stages. Just because training requirements have been met does not mean investigators continue to practice the principles. For example, institutions and funding agencies could assess and report whether trainees are actually conducting experiments that incorporate the four items recommended by Landis. Silberberg said the NIH peer-review process now requires investigators to discuss the rigor of the prior research they are citing as key support of their application. As researchers often cite their own prior work, this necessitates that they acknowledge the shortcomings. He reiterated that research is cyclical, and researchers will come to understand that it is to their advantage to conduct rigorous studies that they can then cite in their next grant application. Carrasquillo emphasized the need for accountability, and proposed a quantitative approach, with the results taken into account in funding renewal and promotion evaluations. For example, investigators could be required to report what percentage of a laboratory's studies included blinding, inclusion–exclusion criteria, randomization, and sample size calculation, and could note the reason why an element might not have been done for a particular study. Silberberg noted the limitations of a quantitative approach, for example, not all experiments can or should be blinded, and the quantitative aspect is lost once investigators can offer an explanation for each study that does not comply. He added that different standards would need to apply to exploratory versus hypothesis testing or confirmatory studies. Coller pointed to the importance of mentorship and the need to take into account "the subtle distinctions" that do not fit into a cell on a spreadsheet, but that are important in the evaluation process. Goodman proposed evaluating scientists and institutions at both ends of the performance spectrum, "not just on their best research, but by their worst." In other words, he elaborated, it would be important to acknowledge when an investigator's "worst" research is still of high quality. If there were some quantification, it would be understood that some research would likely fall at the bottom of the quality scale. However, a few high-impact studies would not balance an overall portfolio of "ignorable" work, he said.

Macleod said the EQIPD project is developing a quality management system that will allow laboratories to self-evaluate, implement measures to improve performance (e.g., designate a quality improvement champion, develop a strategy), and self-assert that their performance is in compliance with the requirements of the scheme. A laboratory will then have a badge as evidence of their performance level, which can be used when applying for grants, submitting manuscripts, or recruiting, for example. The system will be open source and will link supporting resources, including templates.

Training in Systematic Review

Goodman suggested that trainees and young investigators need to be empowered with the skills to conduct methodologic meta-research. Journal clubs, he said, can be an opportunity to identify methods that could be systematically reviewed in depth. This would give students an opportunity to potentially publish a paper, but it also allows them to contribute to improving methodology in their own field, he said. Students become "sensitized to the weaknesses" in the literature in their field and are empowered and motivated to contribute to change. Macleod said the doctoral program in neuroscience at the University of Edinburgh is doing this by having small groups of students conduct a systematic review of the models they will use in their laboratory research. He shared an example of a student who had then applied this in her work.

A participant from the NIH Division of Biomedical Research Workforce said that changes are forthcoming in 2020 that are designed to ensure that NIH training grants include resources for training in rigor, reproducibility, and data science.

Reporting Metadata

Anne Plant, a fellow at the National Institute of Standards and Technology, emphasized the importance of recording and reporting metadata to help deal with the uncertainty around the data. "A measurement consists of two things," she said, "a value ... and the uncertainty around that value." There is uncertainty in each step of the research process, and while steps can be taken to reduce uncertainty, it is never eliminated. Reporting the metadata as well as the meta-analyses, and actions taken to reduce the uncertainty in the data that are collected and reported, allows researchers to "know what is known," and with what level of confidence. Coller pointed out using an electronic notebook provides version control and audit trails and suggested that notebooks could be made available as supplementary material to a publication. Plant said researchers need a tool that would allow them to easily capture and collate all of the metadata around their protocol in real time, not after the fact.

Including Other Stakeholders

Coller prompted participants to consider other stakeholders that should be included in the discussions of transparency and reproducibility. He asked whether a checklist might help those who report on scientific advances to be "better informed about how they write about science," or whether a checklist could help the general public better judge the quality and understand the uncertainties of the many studies in the news.

The Press

Macleod mentioned that the UK government inquiries into the practices of the British Press included inquiries into press coverage of scientific issues. Reports about what causes or cures a disease one day often contradict what was reported the previous day. During the inquiry, Macleod said, it was found that the content of news articles was often taken directly from press releases issued by research institutions. While there are issues to be addressed regarding press coverage of scientific information, he said much of the responsibility for what is reported in the press lies directly with research institutions.

Biomedical Research Investors

Macleod suggested that another stakeholder group in need of quality information about biomedical research is investors. "Those that invest in our pharmaceutical industry are completely uninformed, unaware, and unconcerned about the quality of the biomedical research endeavor," he said. Referring to his earlier example of NXY-059, which was effective in animal models but failed in a large clinical trial, he said that the manufacturer's share price fell by 17 percent, a value of $9.6 billion, over the 2 days after publication of the study results, and it took 7 years to recover.

The Pharmaceutical Industry

Silberberg said another stakeholder is the pharmaceutical industry. He noted that the EQIPD project is a good example of how academia and industry can work together to share data, resources, and expertise to advance product development.

Public Health

Gardenier identified public health as another community with a stake in the quality of biomedical research. Caregivers, community hospital groups, nursing homes, and others in public health administer the benefits of biomedical research to the public.

Evaluating Quality Initiatives

Macleod stressed the importance of evaluating research quality initiatives to show that an intervention is achieving the intended outcome. Depending on the type of intervention, a manufacturing process control chart could be used to monitor change, or a randomized controlled trial might be needed to determine benefit. A challenge, he said, is that vocabulary and methodology do not yet exist for this type of "research on research." He noted the need to proceed cautiously and in a scientific way when "demanding our colleagues and peers change their practice"—he suggested developing the science and methodology and collecting evidence of the impact of interventions to effect lasting change to research practice.

6

Toward Minimal Reporting Standards for Preclinical Biomedical Research

Highlights of Key Points Made by Individual Speakers

- Separate reviewers for different sections (e.g., statistics, methods) could be an approach to share the burden of peer review. (Kolber, Silberberg)
- Grant reviewers could evaluate the reproducibility or adherence to guidelines of primary literature cited in a research proposal, perhaps motivating applicants to more carefully consider the rigor of the studies they reference. (Nakamura)
- The research community and publishers should work collaboratively toward culture change. One issue to be addressed is the addition of underpowered in vivo studies in response to peer-review requests, which can impact the quality of an otherwise compelling paper. (Vinson)
- Many of the tools that support reproducible research are already available through institutional libraries (e.g., data sharing, checklists, preregistration, preprints, sharing code, sharing data, incentives, metrics), and existing research support staff are available to provide expert assistance. (Rethlefsen, Sayre)
- A commonality of successful guidelines is that they facilitate team science, which brings together investigators, collaborators, and research support staff to share the workload. (Sayre)

- Transparent reporting should show "the chain of precise induction," that a method used or chosen is applicable to the problem being solved. Data science tools are available to share relevant information, including the logic and reasoning that were applied during the study analysis. (Keiser)
- Technical solutions (e.g., checklists, minimal reporting standards) can serve as reminders, but they are not sufficient for solving adaptive sociocultural problems and do not substitute for knowledge and understanding. (Goodman)
- "Improving research practices must be driven by scientists reforming their own fields with the help of experts in rigor and reproducibility, impelled by institutional leadership, manifest by structures and metrics." (Goodman)

As the workshop progressed, the discussions transitioned from examining the current state of transparency in preclinical biomedical research to describing opportunities for action (see Box 6-1 for corresponding workshop objectives). Panelists offered their reflections on the workshop thus far and discussed potential stakeholder actions to harmonize guidelines and develop minimal reporting standards.

Benedict Kolber, associate professor at Duquesne University, shared his perspective on what transparent reporting means for reviewers of grants and manuscripts. Richard Nakamura, retired director of the Center for Scientific Review at the National Institutes of Health (NIH), discussed some of the opportunities to review research for reproducibility, and shared several points to keep in mind moving forward. Valda Vin-

BOX 6-1
Workshop Session Objectives

- Discuss opportunities for improving the consistency of reporting guidelines and requirements for rigor and transparency by journals, funders, and institutions across the biomedical research life cycle.
- Consider approaches to compare reporting of rigor elements proposed in grant applications to those included in publications.
- Suggest stakeholder actions to encourage transparent reporting and practical next steps toward establishing minimal reporting standards for preclinical biomedical research.

SOURCE: Workshop agenda (available in Appendix C), September 25 and 26, 2019.

son discussed some of the challenges that journals face as a stakeholder promoting culture change. Franklin Sayre, STEM Librarian at Thompson Rivers University, emphasized the value of engaging research support staff, including librarians, in efforts to increase reproducibility. Melissa Rethlefsen, associate dean, George A. Smathers Libraries and Fackler Director, Health Science Center Libraries at the University of Florida, expanded on the discussion of librarians as partners in leveraging existing resources and driving change within institutions. Michael Keiser, assistant professor at the University of California, San Francisco, shared lessons from developing and testing machine learning models that could be applied to designing and implementing transparent reporting strategies. Steven Goodman discussed the Patient-Centered Outcomes Research Institute (PCORI) Methodology Standards as a case example of an effort to develop minimal standards for the design, conduct, analysis, and reporting of research and the limitations of checklists in changing behavior.

WHAT TRANSPARENT REPORTING MEANS FOR REVIEWERS

Benedict Kolber, Associate Professor, Duquesne University

"Transparency will be the legacy of this rigor, reproducibility, transparency movement," Kolber said. Bad science will happen, and the key is to be transparent and honest about what was done. Moving toward better experimental design is important, he said, but reporting guidelines can be implemented to improve transparency now, regardless of how an experiment was designed. Kolber shared his perspective as an academic researcher and faculty member on what transparent reporting means for reviewers of grants and manuscripts.

Grant Reviewer for a Funder

Guidelines provided by funders to grant reviewers vary widely, Kolber said. He reiterated the point by Shai Silberberg that some review processes now require applicants to discuss the rigor of the data on which they are basing their proposal. Kolber said that as a grant reviewer, however, he often believes he needs to decide how much weight he should give to elements of rigor.

Kolber suggested a starting point could be for NIH to add a rigor attachment to grant applications that is similar to the authentication attachment. NIH requires grant applicants to attach a document describing how chemical and biological resources included in the proposal will be authenticated. This information is not taken into account in scoring, he noted. He suggested that an attachment requiring discussion of the rigor of the experimental design could be added, and initially not included in scoring, to inform discussion of how grant reviewers could evaluate rigor in funding proposals.

Manuscript Peer Reviewer

As mentioned earlier, as transparency in reporting improves and more information is provided in manuscripts, the burden on the reviewers increases, Kolber said. "Reviewers are the last gatekeepers" of scientific quality and being a reviewer has become increasingly more difficult and time intensive as reviewers must apply checklists and review detailed methods. This is essential, but Kolber said that other mechanisms are needed to keep from overburdening peer reviewers.

One approach could be having separate reviewers for different sections. Kolber noted that having separate reviewers for statistics has been suggested. He said a separate reviewer could assess the methods against a checklist before the manuscript is sent to the other reviewers, allowing them to then focus on reviewing the rest of the content for what was done well and what might be missing.

IMPROVING ASSESSMENT OF REPRODUCIBILITY

Richard Nakamura, Former Director of the Center for Scientific Review, National Institutes of Health

Several factors have negatively impacted reproducibility in recent years, Nakamura said. As background, he said that after the congressional effort to double the total NIH budget over the course of 5 years[1] ended in 2003, "all of science in the United States underwent somewhat of a recession." As a result, grant success rates were low and cuts to grant funding were high. This meant, he explained, that researchers had less money for each study, and looked for ways to "cut corners." In addition, he said that researchers continue to face "long and busy waits for research grants, protocol approval, and publication." He also noted that there is "intense pressure" for both researchers and journal editors to improve performance metrics. For example, editors are often rewarded for actions that increase the impact factor of the journal.

---

[1] See detailed information about NIH appropriations at https://www.nih.gov/about-nih/what-we-do/nih-almanac/appropriations-section-1 (accessed February 19, 2020).

Opportunities to Review Research for Reproducibility

Nakamura listed some of the opportunities to review research for reproducibility or for adherence to guidelines or checklists. One approach, he said, would be to redraft grant applications as protocols, which could then be judged for reproducibility, but this approach is not widely preferred by the scientific community. Another opportunity is during protocol review by an Institutional Review Board or an Animal Care and Use Committee. As discussed, however, there are concerns about the impact of increasing the burden on reviewers on the timeliness of approvals.

For the review of grant applications, a general strategy is to have the Principal Investigator commit to follow a set of guidelines (e.g., Consolidated Standards of Reporting Trials [CONSORT]). Another opportunity, Nakamura said, is to have grant reviewers evaluate the reproducibility or adherence to guidelines of the published papers cited in support of the proposed research. To understand the potential impact of this increased burden on reviewers, the Center for Scientific Review surveyed reviewers about the extent to which they look at the primary literature cited by grant applicants. Nakamura said that 90 percent of reviewers responded that they had checked the original papers cited. This suggests that the imposition would be minimal, he said, and researchers might be motivated to more carefully consider the rigor of the publications they cite in grant applications if they know reviewers are taking this into account.

Another opportunity for review of reproducibility and adherence to guidelines is, as discussed, peer and editor review for publication by journals. Nakamura agreed with the comments made that the responsibility does not rest solely with journals. Nonetheless, journal publishers, and particularly high-impact journal publishers, "play a critical role in ensuring that strong papers are the ones that get published," he said.

Moving Forward

Nakamura made several points to keep in mind in moving forward with developing minimum standards for reporting. First, he supported the use of guidelines and checklists and underscored the need to coordinate guidelines for efficiency, and to prioritize the most important checklist items as discussed by Silberberg. He also underscored the need to "keep funding and publication space available for exploratory, discovery, and replication studies." Awarding funding only for protocols will impact exploration and creative ideas. He added that exploratory studies should be transparently reported so that the limitations are clear. Nakamura concurred with Macleod that the impact of interventions on the science ecosystem must be assessed. "Explicit measures of success" are needed, he said, such as workload, cost, and replicability of important findings.

CULTURE CHANGE FOR JOURNAL PUBLISHERS

Valda Vinson, Editor of Research, Science

Much of the workshop discussions focused on the need for culture change in scientific research, so Vinson reflected on the need for culture change within scientific publishing as well. Two decades ago, as an associate editor, it was instilled in Vinson that the scientific community set the standard, and publishers upheld the standard. Journals did not lead, she said; they followed the norms set by the research community. However, as discussed by Brian Nosek (see Chapter 3), all stakeholders contribute to effecting cultural change. She said the research community and publishers need to "be very mindful of one another" in working collaboratively toward change.

In reflecting on the discussions thus far, Vinson highlighted the idea that science is cyclical and cumulative. Journals strive to publish those papers that they believe will allow science to move forward, Vinson said. The primary goal of a journal is "the communication of science to scientists." She recalled that some of the discussions called for journals to change how they decide what to publish. If there is agreement that the overarching goal of a journal is to disseminate high-value scientific information to a broad readership, then a question for discussion, she said, is whether journals are publishing the right research. She also observed that exploratory and confirmatory research are often discussed in the context of one being better or worse than the other, and she suggested different terminology might also be needed for culture change.

Thinking specifically about papers published by her journal, *Science,* Vinson observed that additional studies done in response to a reviewer, as a condition of publication, are often underpowered and of lower quality. A resubmitted manuscript might have three figures showing data from well-powered in vitro studies, for example, and a fourth figure with new data from an underpowered in vivo study, because a reviewer comment said that the paper should include in vivo data. The resubmitted manuscript then meets the reviewer's requirement. Vinson suggested that changes to the publishing culture should be done in partnership with the research community. Vinson said this type of culture change could evolve in the publishing community, but not without the same culture change within the research community (i.e., with support from reviewers and researchers).

ENGAGING RESEARCH SUPPORT STAFF

Franklin Sayre, STEM Librarian, Thompson Rivers University

Basic and clinical researchers are supported by a cadre of research support staff, including statisticians, computer scientists, librarians, archivists, and others. Sayre shared his perspective as a science, technology, engineering, and mathematics (STEM) librarian supporting evidence-based medicine. He pointed out that many of the issues related to reproducibility involve "scholarly communication" (e.g., data sharing, checklists, preregistration, preprints, code sharing, incentives, metrics). The research support community and research libraries have expertise to contribute to the discussions on these issues.

As a STEM librarian, Sayre said that he regularly works with graduate students and postdoctoral fellows who are seeking guidance on how to implement a required checklist, or who are interested in designing reproducible research. He described his role as happening within a "black box" that sits among research policy, incentives, and infrastructure on one side, and reproducible, rigorous research on the other. He said research support staff and the work they do in that black box are often missing from the conversations about reproducibility.

Sayre considered why there has not been more uptake of rigorous and reproducible research methodologies. Guidelines and checklists are available, as well as tools and infrastructure, such as open source frameworks and data repositories. He said what may be needed is not more repositories, but rather, better funding and support for existing resources. Sayre noted that the researchers he has worked with often believe that using checklists early in the research process gives them confidence that they are not missing something that will impact their ability to publish. He suggested that one reason for the lack of uptake, as has been discussed, is the current incentive structure. Another reason is that designing reproducible research can be complicated as it may require knowledge and technical skill in areas of scholarly communication, such as programming, data sharing, data curation, research policy, checklists, guidelines, preregistration, and publishing issues.

Sayre also considered what lessons can be learned from the successful implementation of reporting guidelines such as Preferred Reporting Items for Systematic Reviews and Meta-Analyses (PRISMA) and CONSORT.[2] He suggested that one commonality of successful guidelines is that they facilitate team science, bringing together investigators, collaborators, and research support staff, and sharing the burden.

Workshop participants previously raised the idea of creating a new profession to fill the black box, but Sayre pointed out that most institutions already have "a constellation of experts" who can advise on study design, statistical analysis, data management (e.g., curation, repositories, sharing), policies, and other elements of reproducible research. These

[2] Brief background information on selected guidelines, including PRISMA and CONSORT, is available in Appendix B.

experts work within departments, computing centers, and libraries, for example. In closing, Sayre said that research support staff should establish an identity as a stakeholder group so they are included in the discussions about enabling reproducibility in biomedical research and can contribute to solutions.

LIBRARIANS DRIVING INSTITUTIONAL CHANGE

Melissa Rethlefsen, Associate Dean, George A. Smathers Libraries, and Fackler Director, Health Science Center Libraries, University of Florida

"Institutions drive the publish or perish, funding or famine culture," said Rethlefsen, and they play a role in changing that culture and promoting reproducibility of research. Although lack of reproducibility and transparency is of particular concern to the field of preclinical biomedical research, all disciplines, even the humanities, face problems with reproducibility of research.

Institutions should find ways to help researchers succeed, Rethlefsen said, and one approach may be to engage libraries and librarians as partners. As Sayre mentioned, librarians have expertise in scholarly communications and understand the research life cycle. Librarians are transdisciplinary, skilled at working with faculty, staff, and students in all disciplines, including researchers, educators, and clinicians. Many of the tools to support reproducible research are already available through institutional libraries, she said, such as institutional repositories, and support for data management and data curation. In addition, libraries are "natural partners" with other research resources such as the institutional Office of Research, Clinical and Translational Science Awards Program Hubs, high-performance computing centers, and biostatistics cores. Rethlefsen described two case examples that illustrate how librarians are helping to drive institutional change by serving as faculty members and by leveraging tools and services and supporting curricular integration, professional development, advocacy and outreach, and coalition building.

University of Utah

While working at the University of Utah, Rethlefsen became aware that the vice president for research was interested in the reproducibility of preclinical research and it was decided that the library would plan and host a research reproducibility conference in 2016. The conference explored ways in which the library could support reproducibility of research, including leveraging existing resources and relationships. For example, the library had partnered with the Center for Clinical and Translational Science at the university to establish a systematic review core, and the library had supported an event raising awareness of sex and gender differences in research. The convergence of these and other resources (e.g., the Study Design and Biostatistics Core) enabled the library to support more rigorous research in general and to assist with addressing rigor and reproducibility in preparing grant applications. As awareness of the library's resources for reproducibility grew, Rethlefsen said librarians were asked to teach classes, assist with lectures, and develop partnerships. For example, she said the library helped to establish the university's first JupyterHub server to teach reproducible Python scripting. The library was asked to teach the reproducibility sessions of the DeCart summer program in biomedical data science and teaches part of the Research Administration Training Series.

Rethlefsen said that feedback after the 2016 conference indicated that stakeholders across disciplines were eager to connect in a neutral forum such as the library. This illustrates the importance of grassroots initiatives. The library continues to scale its efforts and has launched a Grand Rounds Reproducibility Series (a weekly lecture on reproducibility in research in different disciplines) and an interdisciplinary Research Reproducibility Coalition to push for policy change at the institutional level. A second Research Reproducibility Conference was held in 2018, designed specifically to teach researchers the skills needed for reproducible research, including working with reporting guidelines and minimum reporting standards.

University of Florida

At the University of Florida, where Rethlefsen currently works, she is deploying the same strategy to identify existing resources, establish partnerships, and drive change. One existing library resource is the Academic Research Consulting and Services group, which has a data management librarian, informatics and bioinformatics librarians, a clinical and translational science institute liaison librarian, and a research impact librarian. To more effectively support reproducibility and reduce the burden on researchers, the library is hiring new faculty, including a reproducibility librarian, and, in partnership with the university's Clinical and Translational Science Institute, a systematic review librarian.

As before, Rethlefsen said, library faculty are also involved in teaching, curriculum development (e.g., rigor and reproducibility training as required by NIH training grants), and professional development (e.g., how to use Python, Open Science Framework, reporting guidelines). The library collaborated with Research Computing at the university to host a Research Bazaar, which is a worldwide event to promote digital literacy.

Planning is under way for a research reproducibility conference in 2020, she said, that will focus on best practices for education about research reproducibility.

In closing, Rethlefsen said there are existing resources and practices, some of which may be grassroots efforts, which can be leveraged by institutions. She emphasized that sustaining grassroots or "volunteer" efforts is challenging, and support from institutional leadership is needed for success.

APPLYING A SYSTEMATIC FRAMEWORK TO DEVELOPING MIMIMAL REPORTING STANDARDS

Michael Keiser, Assistant Professor, University of California, San Francisco

Keiser shared his perspective on transparent reporting as an early career researcher, drawing on Platt's systematic and transparent approach to science, which Platt termed "strong inference"—a model of inquiry that relies on alternative hypotheses rather than a single hypothesis to avoid bias (Platt, 1964). Keiser described an example of Platt's approach which, while systematic, allows for creativity and exploration (see Figure 6-1). The approach begins with devising a hypothesis and a set of alternative hypotheses—feasible and falsifiable statements that can be tested experimentally. The second step is to design one or more experiments to disprove or exclude one or more of the hypotheses. Platt's third step is to conduct the experiments. This three-step process is then refined and repeated until only one hypothesis remains. Keiser cautioned that measurements (e.g., numbers, statistics, calculations) can be misleading depending on how they are framed. There is also the risk that researchers may substitute correlation with causation. Keiser emphasized that a hypothesis can never be proven or confirmed, but it can certainly be disproven.

With this as background, Keiser then transitioned to application of strong inference toward machine learning. "We must be our own adversaries to the models we develop," Keiser said. He described controls for use in computational sciences (including machine learning) that he said could be applied more broadly to data science and analysis (Chuang and Keiser, 2018).

First, Keiser argued that there is no black box for computational models. There are techniques to investigate computational models and, similar to other types of research, it is important to ask whether the model is logical. As an example, Keiser described one of his own studies using machine learning to detect the presence of different types of amyloid

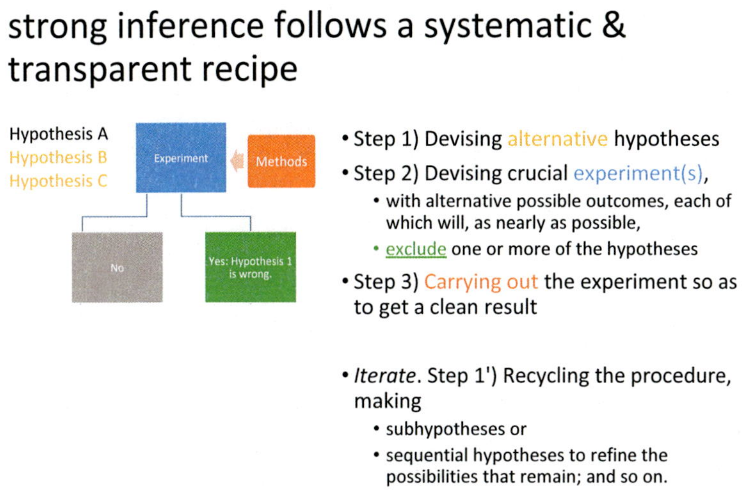

FIGURE 6-1 Strong inference follows a systematic and transparent recipe, consisting of iterating from hypotheses and alternative hypotheses through devising and conducting crucial experiments in a replicable manner until all possible hypotheses are evaluated and only one remains.
SOURCES: Keiser presentation, September 26, 2019; citing Platt in *Science*, 1964.

plaques in the brains of deceased Alzheimer's disease patients (Tang et al., 2019). Keiser explained how his team trained a neural network to rapidly classify plaques (e.g., diffuse or cored) based on image analysis. Keiser added that a preprint of the paper was posted on bioRxiv and the data were posted to the open access repository, Zenodo. This study had already been replicated by others using different datasets before the paper was accepted for publication.

When considering minimal reporting standards, Keiser suggested applying Platt's strong inference approach when choosing scientific methods that are appropriate for a given problem. Transparent reporting should include information on the logic and reasoning that went into a study analysis, he said. Data science tools are already available to encode and share relevant information, including preregistration in Registered Reports, software version control using Git, data repositories through Zenodo, and logic models using Jupyter notebook.

In closing, Keiser said researchers should be their own adversaries. Drawing on lessons from the field of cybersecurity: a "red team" is a group of good actors tasked with attacking digital infrastructure to test an organization's defenses. Keiser suggested that one approach for the biomedical field could be to establish a similar type of a red team within research groups or institutions in which scientists perform regular checks on each other's work. Perhaps this could be a potential research support career path.

THE IMPACT OF MINIMAL STANDARDS ON IMPROVING METHODOLOGY

Steven Goodman, Professor of Medicine and Health Research and Policy and Co-Director of METRICS, Stanford University

Goodman briefly shared his perspective as a research educator on some of the critical gaps in the training of research scientists. Many laboratory scientists, early career as well as some senior investigators, have a limited understanding of the "basic elements and formal logic and purpose of experimental design," he said, including blinding, randomization, sample size determination, and other aspects. Laboratory scientists often have limited training in the "foundations of statistical inference and the meaning of basic statistical summaries," he continued. Reiterating his comment from earlier in the workshop, he said that doctoral students are often enrolled in advanced analysis courses without understanding the concepts covered in introductory courses. Many researchers do not understand the links among "the question, the design, the measurements, the conduct, the analysis, the inference, the conclusions, and the generalizations" in the chain of experimentation, he said. Lastly, he said that "virtually every gap in training or understanding is created or reinforced by the literature they read." He asserted that it is extremely challenging to train new scientists to conduct rigorous science when that is not what they are seeing published in high-profile journals.

PCORI Methodology Standards

Goodman discussed the PCORI Methodology Standards as a case example of an effort to develop minimal standards for the design, conduct, analysis, and reporting of research. The law authorizing PCORI mandated the establishment of a Methodology Committee and the development of methodology standards for patient-centered outcomes research by the committee, with input from stakeholders and the public.[3] The standards are used to assess the rigor of studies proposed in funding applications received by PCORI, and to monitor the conduct and reporting of funded

[3] Further information about PCORI's methodology research, including the PCORI Methodology Report, and the members of the Methodology Committee, is available at https://www.pcori.org/research-results/about-our-research/research-methodology (accessed November 20, 2019).

studies, Goodman said.[4] A total of 65 standards for patient-centered outcomes research were developed in 16 topic areas, including 5 cross-cutting areas and 11 for specific elements of research (see Box 6-2).

Goodman listed the four Standards for Preventing and Handling Missing Data (MD) and provided excerpts from the explanation of the second standard (PCORI, 2019):

- "MD-1: Describe methods to prevent and monitor missing data."
- "MD-2: Use valid statistical methods to deal with missing data that properly account for statistical uncertainty due to missingness.... Estimates of treatment effects or measures of association should ... account for statistical uncertainty attributable to missing data. Methods used for imputing missing data should produce valid confidence intervals and permit unbiased inferences.... *Single imputation methods, such as last observation carried forward, baseline*

BOX 6-2
Patient-Centered Outcomes Research Institute (PCORI) Methodology Standards Topic Areas

Cross-Cutting Standards
- Formulating Research Questions
- Patient-Centeredness
- Data Integrity and Rigorous Analyses
- Preventing and Handling Missing Data
- Heterogeneity of Treatment Effects

Design-Specific Standards
- Data Registries
- Data Networks
- Causal Inference Methods
- Adaptive and Bayesian Trial Designs
- Studies of Medical Tests
- Systematic Reviews
- Research Designs Using Clusters
- Studies of Complex Interventions
- Qualitative Methods
- Mixed Methods Research
- Individual Participant-Level Data Meta-Analysis (IPD-MA)

SOURCES: Goodman presentation, September 26, 2019; adapted from PCORI, 2019.

[4] The current Methodology Standards are available at https://www.pcori.org/methodology-standards (accessed November 20, 2019).

observation carried forward, and mean value imputation, are discouraged…" [emphasis Goodman].
- "MD-3: Record and report all reasons for dropout and missing data, and account for all patients in reports."
- "MD-4: Examine sensitivity of inferences to missing data methods and assumptions and incorporate into interpretation."

"These are basic principles" and seem relatively "minimal and obvious," Goodman said. However, they are not necessarily easy to assess. As an example, he challenged participants to consider exactly how they might assess compliance with the standard that reads, "Single imputation methods, such as last observation carried forward, baseline observation carried forward, and mean value imputation, are discouraged." He added that assessing applicable standards can require "a fair amount of sophisticated judgment."

The adherence of final reports to the PCORI Methodology Standards was evaluated and presented at the Eighth International Congress on Peer Review and Scientific Publication (Mayo-Wilson et al., 2017). None of the 31 final reports assessed had adhered to all of the standards, Goodman reported. He highlighted that "many reports did not use appropriate methods for handling missing data," and "most reports examined heterogeneity with subgroup analyses, but few studies conducted confirmatory tests for heterogeneity." This shows that simply having the standards in place was not sufficient, Goodman said. He observed that although PCORI "has substantial leverage and resources" as a funder, it still faces challenges in influencing practice. PCORI is now conducting a portfolio review of applications and final reports to determine if potential issues in final reports can be detected and prevented early. He added that it is much more difficult to implement true policy solutions that change practice than to develop technical solutions (i.e., standards).

Implications of a "Simple Checklist"

Goodman read excerpts from a 2009 commentary by Pronovost and colleagues on the interest in and implications of the checklist intervention Pronovost developed in 2006 to reduce central line infections in the Michigan Keystone ICU program.[5] The checklist was hailed in the media as a simple solution to a serious patient safety problem. According to Pronovost and colleagues, however, "the mistake of the 'simple checklist' story is in the assumption that a technical solution (checklists) can solve

[5] The original article describing the intervention is available at https://www.nejm.org/doi/full/10.1056/NEJMoa061115 (accessed November 20, 2019).

an adaptive (sociocultural) problem" (Bosk et al., 2009, p. 444). Goodman emphasized two sections of the commentary for participants to reflect on as they considered the development and implementation of guidelines.

- "Widespread deployment of checklists without an appreciation for how or why they work is a potential threat to patients' safety and high-quality care" (Bosk et al., 2009, p. 444).
- "Indeed, it would be a mistake to say there was one 'Keystone checklist.' There was not a uniform instrument, but rather, more than 100 versions" (Bosk et al., 2009, p. 445).

Goodman summarized that technical solutions (e.g., checklists, minimal reporting standards) can serve as reminders, but they are not sufficient for solving adaptive sociocultural problems and do not substitute for knowledge or understanding. In the absence of knowledge and understanding, enforcing minimal reporting standards may require significant effort and produce limited results. "Pressure and legitimacy need to be exerted at all levels, from funders, journals, regulators, and professional societies, but change has to occur on the ground level, and must include education and the means to operationalize it," Goodman said. "Improving research practices must be driven by scientists reforming their own fields with the help of experts in rigor and reproducibility, impelled by institutional leadership, manifest by structures and metrics," he added. He emphasized the importance of partnering with sociologists and organizational experts who study institutional and disciplinary change.

DISCUSSION

Increasing Rigor and Enhancing Transparency

Harvey Fineberg observed that the some of the suggestions raised during the workshop discussions were specific to increasing scientific rigor, while others focused on enhancing transparency, and some suggestions covered the intersection of the two. He noted the need to keep both the distinctions and connections between rigor and transparency in mind when discussing potential solutions for improving reproducibility and the roles of stakeholders, including researchers, institutions, funders, publishers/editors, and the larger scientific community.

Shai Silberberg said that, in his opinion, rigor and transparency are the same in the sense that transparency leads to rigor. Alexa McCray agreed and said that "transparency and rigor are two sides of the same coin" and that being transparent from the start, and transparent throughout, can reduce the burdens associated with reproducibility because transparency facilitates assessment by the broader scientific community. The benefits of openness and transparency are discussed in the National Academies consensus study report *Open Science by Design*, McCray said (NASEM, 2018).

Arturo Casadevall agreed that, while transparency can promote rigor, the two concepts are distinct, as discussed by Fineberg. Highly rigorous science can be conducted in secrecy (i.e., without transparency), as might be done for military weapons research, for example. However, transparency can "promote rigor, independently of the tenants that define rigor," he said.

Goodman countered that rigor and transparency are inextricable in that "we can't trust science that we can't see." Science must be transparent to be convincing. Science that is rigorous, but not transparent, is often not reproducible or translatable and, in the absence of confirmation, does not lead to a consensus among scientists of what might be considered "fact" or "truth."

Kolber observed that definitions for reproducibility and replicability had been discussed earlier in the workshop, but transparency as it applies to research reporting had not been fully defined. He encouraged participants to consider what would be required to develop a fully transparently reported manuscript. Deborah Sweet suggested that involving trainees and postdoctoral fellows in the review process would be helpful given that they are the scientists who are actually carrying out the laboratory experiments and therefore best suited to determine if there is sufficient information provided in a manuscript to allow them to reproduce or replicate the study.

Addressing Underpowered In Vivo Studies

Thomas Curran asserted that it is "unethical to conduct a bad animal experiment." He reiterated a point made several times during the workshop that researchers may add an underpowered animal study or use an inappropriate animal model in response to a request by a peer reviewer. He called on journal editors to intervene when reviewers ask for such studies. Vinson responded that journals do not intentionally publish animal studies that are underpowered or are done in inappropriate models, but editors rely on the reviewers, who are the experts. She observed that there is now increased awareness of this issue and that journals are implementing statistical reviews to establish thresholds for publication of such studies.

Nosek suggested that one approach to addressing this issue could be for journals not to require additional in vivo studies for publication. Nosek suggested that this could be an opportunity to use Registered Reports—a publishing format in which protocols are provisionally accepted for publication regardless of whether the result is positive or negative if the authors follow through with the registered methodology. Authors who are asked by reviewers to conduct additional experiments could submit a study design and protocol to Registered Reports, which the journal would review and commit to publish the results. This approach would help alleviate pressure on the researcher to generate a positive result for publication, Nosek said. Furthermore, he suggested that a journal could compare current practice to this approach to determine whether the intervention has an impact on reproducibility of results. Vinson added that this type of randomized assessment would likely require participation of more than one journal.

Considering Peer Review

Silberberg observed that publication in high-profile journals often requires that manuscripts include a host of different techniques to address a scientific question from multiple angles. He added that it is unrealistic to expect a single investigator to have such broad expertise, which is why many of the studies published in high-profile journals are collaborations. The result is that some authors may not fully understand all of the content in a given manuscript or may not be able to critically evaluate the contributions of other authors. More importantly, Silberberg continued, reviewers may not have the breadth of expertise to critically evaluate the entirety of a manuscript. He shared that during the National Institute of Neurological Disorders and Stroke stakeholder workshop held in 2012 (see Landis et al., 2012), participants discussed the approach of enlisting multiple reviewers with expertise in different domains. Another approach, he suggested, would be for journals to allow publication of manuscripts that are more narrowly focused. He described a case example in which a paper in a high-profile journal was retracted due to concerns about a single image in a panel of dozens. He postulated that the image, related to an animal experiment, may have been added in response to peer review.

Conducting Reproducibility and Replicability Studies

Kolber said investigators are focused on discovery, and "the idea of replicating another finding is not interesting." He noted that small replication studies to bring a new model into the laboratory are common and are not generally published, even if they fail. Keiser added that, currently, if a researcher finds a problem in a published paper, they might contact the author about the disagreement, publish a commentary piece, or engage in other types of public back-and-forth discussion, all of which takes a lot of effort and a long time. Perhaps there could be support for finding problems of irreproducibility, somewhat similar to the "bug bounties" used to identify security vulnerabilities in technology products and services, he said. He suggested that training grants could cover attempts by trainees to reproduce studies in their field of research and could even require it as a way to enhance training in rigorous research.

7

Stakeholder Opportunities for Promoting Transparent Reporting

For the final session of the workshop, participants broke into small groups to consider the roles and responsibilities of researchers, publishers, institutions, and funders in improving transparent reporting of biomedical research.

In preparation for the small group activity, Harvey Fineberg shared his impressions from the workshop presentations and discussions thus far. There is simultaneously readiness and reluctance to act on improving transparency, he observed. He noted that ideas and attitudes about transparency seem to be converging in the right direction, and resources are being mobilized. However, he said, there remain "cultural barriers to introducing, implementing, and fulfilling the aspirations of open science through transparency." Tools are available to researchers, publishers, and funders to promote rigorous research and transparent reporting. The task now is to determine what may be missing, what needs to be improved, and how stakeholder needs can be addressed, Fineberg said. During the small group discussions, he asked participants to identify what they consider the most important opportunities for moving forward.

Over the course of the workshop, perspectives were shared by researchers—from early career scientists to senior investigators and research support staff, as well as representatives of publishers, institutions, and funders. Fineberg asked participants to consider how stakeholder interests could be harmonized, and operations aligned, to realize the shared objective of increased transparency and rigor in research. He also asked participants to consider what leadership role each stakeholder plays in driving transparent reporting in biomedical research.

SMALL GROUP DISCUSSION REPORTS[1]

Upon reconvening in plenary session, a facilitator from each small group summarized the individual participants' discussion (a summary of points made by small group participants is provided in Box 7-1). Group discussions were guided by the following prompts:

- What actions should funders, researchers, institutions, and journals take to drive widespread adoption of minimal reporting standards?
- Are reporting categories in guidelines for publishing (e.g., materials, design, analysis, and reporting) relevant for funders? For institutions? For small publishers/professional societies?
- What other information or reporting categories would be relevant?
- How should funders instruct reviewers of grant applications to reinforce transparent reporting? How much information should funders request (i.e., to what level of detail) in grant applications? Is it possible to obtain sufficient information about transparent reporting in grant applications without dramatic expansion of the application?

BOX 7-1
Suggestions by Individual Workshop Participants on Stakeholder Opportunities to Promote Transparent Reporting in Preclinical Biomedical Research

Researchers

- Researchers may help promote adoption of minimal standards for transparency and rigor through a number of actions, including
  - Considering ways to include information regarding the reasoning and decision points that go into a research project, in addition to using a minimal checklist, when submitting research applications to funders or manuscripts to journals; and
  - Considering ways to leverage the expertise of university librarians and create resources for investigators starting a new laboratory (e.g., look to concepts such as the University of California's QB3 "startup in a box" framework—a combination of hands-on support, services, and mentorship—which is designed to lower the barriers to innovation for university entrepreneurs interested in starting a company).

[1] This small group exercise was intended to engage participants in using what they had learned thus far in the workshop. This section of the proceedings summarizes the small group discussions based on the report by each group's designated rapporteur and should not be construed as reflecting any consensus of the group. All group responses and proposals reported are for discussion purposes only.

- Researchers across all career stages have opportunities to take action to promote reproducibility through transparent reporting:
  - Considering ways to facilitate more substantive feedback on proposals, particularly for early-stage research, through peer review—internally within institutions as well as through external grant applications;
  - Incorporating reproducibility and/or replicability studies into graduate training programs (e.g., coursework, qualifying exams); and
  - Promoting a culture of openness and establishing data-sharing best practices within their laboratories.

NOTE: Points made by individual workshop participants discussing the role of researchers in promoting transparent reporting, as reported by Michael Keiser.

Institutions

- Institutions have opportunities to address impediments to transparency and reproducibility, including
  - Clarifying the criteria for tenure and promotion decisions for early-career researchers;
  - Finding ways to incentivize "transparency, openness, contribution to the research corpus, datasets, [and] even being honest about ... negative results" (e.g., awards, performance bonuses, incorporation into training throughout researchers' careers);
  - Reframing practices that promote transparency and reproducibility (e.g., checklists, data sharing) as a routine part of the scientific research process rather than added administrative burden;
  - Identifying and sharing existing research practices that enhance data sharing and transparent reporting;
  - Considering better mechanisms for connecting researchers with institutional resources; and
  - Engaging leadership and on-the-ground researchers to help build momentum at all levels of the institution.

NOTE: Points made by individual workshop participants discussing the role of institutions in promoting transparent reporting, as reported by Franklin Sayre and Deborah Sweet.

Funders

- Funding organizations have opportunities to enhance transparency and reproducibility, including
  - Considering a priority set of core standards based on what is most important for enhancing transparent reporting in biomedical research;
  - Harmonizing a set of minimal reporting standards across funding groups to help reduce the burden on researchers;
  - Supporting training opportunities and the development of tools and platforms that are interoperable across systems;
  - Promoting culture change through leadership at all levels of an organization; and

continued

BOX 7-1 Continued

- Defining metrics for determining whether interventions lead to the intended outcome.

NOTE: Points made by individual workshop participants discussing the role of funders in promoting transparent reporting, as reported by Richard Nakamura.

Publishers

- Publishers (and funders) can help "bookend the process" of promoting transparent reporting through a number of activities, including
  - Working with other stakeholders from across sectors (e.g., funders, researchers, institutions) to harmonize a set of minimal reporting standards to facilitate better science;
  - Aligning reporting requirements with transparent reporting practices so expectations are clear for researchers throughout the biomedical research life cycle;
  - Considering pragmatic and inclusive approaches to implementing interventions, such as checklists; and
  - Helping to coordinate action to address areas of highest need (e.g., study design, statistics, data archiving, sourcing of biological materials).

NOTE: Points made by individual workshop participants discussing the role of publishers in promoting transparent reporting, as reported by Veronique Kiermer and Valda Vinson.

SOURCE: Rapporteurs' summary of the small group facilitators' reports. This summary is based on individual comments made by individual workshop participants and should not be construed as reflecting any consensus of workshop attendees. All suggestions and proposals are reported for discussion purposes only.

Researchers

Michael Keiser reported for a small group that discussed the roles and responsibilities of researchers in improving transparent reporting of biomedical research. The small group discussions focused on potential actions that various stakeholders could take to help promote widespread adoption of minimal standards for transparency and rigor.

The first proposal, Keiser described, would be for researchers to report, in a standardized way, the reasoning and decision points that went into a given research project as well as relevant gaps in information. He acknowledged that few tools exist to facilitate this type of transparent reporting, so the development of new, more dynamic tools may be needed. Keiser suggested that this information should be included instead of or in addition to minimal reporting standards when submitting research applications to funders or manuscripts to journals.

The second proposal, Keiser outlined, would be to leverage the expertise of university librarians and create a resource for investigators starting a new laboratory. This resource might be similar in concept to the University of California's QB3 "startup in a box" framework—a combination of hands-on support, services, and mentorship—which is designed to lower the barriers to innovation for university entrepreneurs interested in starting a company.[2] This type of resource could provide biomedical researchers with a basic set of tools along with guidance on data access and sharing, standardization, compliance, and other information that early stage investigators may need to establish a new lab. Such a resource could also be useful for more senior investigators seeking to implement new tools or approaches.

Keiser shared additional points raised during the small group discussion regarding actions specific to trainees, early career researchers, and senior investigators that could help promote reproducibility and replication.

For trainees, a few participants suggested that reproducibility and replicability could be incorporated into graduate training programs. For example, graduate students, in consultation with faculty mentors, could be required to reproduce or replicate a study as part of their training grant or qualifying exam. Keiser said the feasibility of reproducing a study might vary by discipline, so perhaps a compilation of existing studies for this type of exercise could be a useful resource. Participants in the small group discussions pointed out that aligning training with a desired change in research practice would help support a culture of reproducibility rather than add administrative burden. Additionally, Keiser noted that participants in the small group discussed the value of implementing formal coursework in experimental research design for undergraduates across institutions.

Participants in the small group said that early career researchers may be more directly connected to the research and the data and more comfortable adopting new tools and practices than senior investigators, Keiser reported. Participants suggested that more substantive feedback, particularly for early stage research proposals, through peer review—internally within institutions as well as through external grant applications—would benefit investigators at all stages of their careers.

Finally, Keiser relayed that small group participants discussed the influential role of senior investigators in promoting a culture of openness (e.g., code review within the lab, experimental reproducibility and replicability by others within the group) and data-sharing practices (e.g., open

[2] Available at https://qb3.org/support-for-launch (accessed January 10, 2020).

source tools, preprints, repositories for sharing data with the broader research community).

Institutions

Franklin Sayre and Deborah Sweet reported for the two small groups that discussed ways institutions can help promote research practices that improve transparency and reproducibility.

Sayre laid out a few institutional impediments to transparency and reproducibility, which were raised by small group participants. In particular, he noted that the real and perceived incentives for tenure and promotion decisions do not necessarily align with incentives for transparent reporting. The tenure process can be a source of great anxiety for early career researchers. Participants suggested that this anxiety and focus on particular metrics, such as publication in high-impact journals, may promote a culture of poor research practices. Participants from both small groups discussed the need for more clarity for early career researchers on how tenure and promotion decisions are made at institutions. Sweet added that when funders show they value transparency, institutions will follow, which is why cooperation across stakeholders is critical. Sweet reported that small group participants discussed the possibility of assigning value to transparent reporting and team science. For example, she suggested that institutions could request tenure support letters to address a nominee's "quality of contribution" to the research environment.

Small group participants also discussed how standards for awarding doctoral degrees should not be based on publication of a given number of papers, but should instead reward "transparency, openness, contribution to the research corpus, datasets, [and] even being honest about your negative results," Sweet said. She added that positive incentives for applying best practices in research transparency might include awards (e.g., the National Institute of Neurological Disorders and Stroke's Landis Mentorship Award[3]) or performance bonuses. She highlighted the importance of training doctoral students from the start and providing training to the broader scientific community as well. Training should make researchers aware of the availability of statistical advice and the value of consulting statisticians at the start of the research process. Steven Goodman added that institutions have a responsibility to provide adequate capacity for statistical and computational science support for researchers.

Sayre described another impediment discussed by small group participants, which was the perception that activities to support transparent

[3] Available at https://www.ninds.nih.gov/Funding/About-Funding/landis-award-for-outstanding-mentorship (accessed January 10, 2020).

reporting constitute an administrative burden and that reproducibility studies are separate from the general "conduct of science." Participants highlighted the need to reframe practices that promote transparency and reproducibility (e.g., checklists, data sharing) as a routine part of the scientific research process. Sweet shared a suggestion by small group participants that institutions might consider developing an inventory of existing research practices from across different laboratories to help identify and share approaches for enabling data sharing and transparent reporting. Institutions could then consider ways to incentivize the uptake of best practices, Sweet said, and perhaps create disincentives for not meeting particular research practice standards.

Sayre relayed a third impediment discussed by small group participants, which was the gap between researchers and institution-level policy, incentives, infrastructure, and research support. Participants suggested there is a need for guidance and better mechanisms to connect researchers with institutional resources. Sweet highlighted one main message raised during the small group discussion: the research culture set by leadership matters, and permeates throughout the organization. She added that institutions should create a "culture of openness" in which there are mechanisms for researchers to raise concerns about reproducibility and consequences for noncompliance with transparent reporting. Sayre also acknowledged that institutional leadership is needed to support widespread adoption of transparent reporting. However, he relayed that "[early career] researchers are often more interested in reproducibility, in transparency, and in sharing their work openly." Small group participants discussed how small laboratories or investigators are often the driving force for grassroots change, so engaging these individuals could help build momentum for reproducibility and transparency within institutions. Sweet shared that small group participants raised the importance of approaching issues with transparent reporting from the perspective that most researchers want to "do the right thing and perform science honestly," rather than taking a punitive approach.

Funders

Richard Nakamura reported for a small group that discussed the roles and responsibilities of funders in improving transparent reporting of biomedical research. Participants in the small group considered the benefit of harmonizing a set of minimal reporting standards across organizations so that investigators are not put in a position of having to meet multiple requirements when applying to different funders. Nakamura relayed the consideration that the application of a common set of minimal reporting standards would need to be flexible across organizations. As discussed throughout the workshop, participants in this small group underscored the need to prioritize a core set of standards based on what is most important for enhancing transparent reporting in biomedical research.

Having tools available will be the key to helping facilitate interoperability across systems and reduce the burden on researchers, Nakamura reported. Small group participants pointed out that funders should adapt to support the development of tools and platforms for transparent reporting as well as replication studies.

The small group discussed how funding organizations can play a significant role in promoting culture change. Small group participants emphasized the need for training, Nakamura said. He added that National Institutes of Health training requirements on this topic should be forthcoming. Similar to other small group discussions, participants highlighted the role of leadership, including those at funding organizations, scientific societies, and academia. Department chairs and senior scientists as well as early career scientists will need to speak up about the problems related to reproducibility and replicability and push for culture change.

Finally, Nakamura said the small group discussed the importance of having metrics to measure whether a given approach leads to improvement. He added that there should be a feedback loop to evaluate whether a given intervention leads to the intended outcome.

Publishers

Veronique Kiermer and Valda Vinson reported for two small groups, which considered the roles and responsibilities of publishers in improving transparent reporting of biomedical research. Vinson summarized the takeaway message of one small group discussion by saying, "If you want science better, make better science easier." Kiermer summarized that institutions can help facilitate transparent reporting practices and make them normative, while journals and funders may "bookend the process" by aligning reporting requirements so that expectations are clear for researchers from the beginning.

One key topic discussed by small group participants was the need for coordinated action across sectors to address areas of highest need. One small group focused on study design and statistics, which might benefit from training modules developed for researchers and institutions as well as for journals and funders, Vinson said. Kiermer shared two areas of need discussed by the other small group: data archiving and sourcing biological materials. Data archiving is essential for transparent reporting, Kiermer said, but efforts are not coordinated. Publishers find that researchers reach the publication stage without having considered from the beginning how they intend to store datasets, including images. As reported by Kiermer, small group participants suggested that the research flow could be improved (1) if funders set expectations from the beginning (e.g., requiring a data management plan as a condition of funding; providing guidance); (2) if institutions provided guidance to researchers on developing a data management plan and use of data repositories; and (3) if journals required reporting of raw data, which could help facilitate review or reproducibility studies following publication. Biological materials are also a source of variability in preclinical studies that contribute to the lack of reproducibility, said Kiermer. Small group participants suggested that clear identification of reagents, authentication of biological material, and archiving of reagents in a repository are all ways to help address this issue, Kiermer reported. For example, participants said the MD Anderson Cancer Center requires authentication of cell lines every year and has established a core facility to help carry out this work.

The small groups both discussed practical approaches for harmonizing a set of minimal reporting standards to facilitate better science. Vinson and Kiermer said that as discussed throughout the workshop, small group participants acknowledged that checklists on their own are not a solution—there would need to be a pragmatic and inclusive approach to implementation. Participants suggested that establishing a coordinated framework, which clearly outlines stakeholder expectations (e.g., editors, authors, reviewers, and the public), would help to drive the adoption of interventions, such as checklists, Vinson said. "Less is more" when promoting compliance with checklists, Kiermer added. Participants acknowledged the challenges of tracking compliance and noted the importance of metadata and persistent identifiers for digital objects "so that there is a clear provenance" from grant application to final publication, Kiermer said.

Finally, small group participants emphasized the need for cross-sector leadership and broad sector inclusion, Kiermer relayed. Participants noted the important role of institutional libraries, and the need to include the perspective of researchers. In this regard, Kiermer said that several small group participants supported the establishment of an ongoing National Academies forum as discussed by Marcia McNutt (see Chapter 2). Vinson suggested the concept of a "sea change" initiative to improve reproducibility in biomedical research that could be modeled after the American Association for the Advancement of Science STEM Equity Achievement (SEA)[4] Change initiative on diversity, equity, and inclusion in science, or the Athena Scientific Women's Academic Network (SWAN) Charter[5]

---

[4] Available at https://seachange.aaas.org (accessed January 10, 2020).

[5] Available at https://www.ecu.ac.uk/equality-charters/athena-swan (accessed January 10, 2020).

promoting gender equity in science in the United Kingdom. In essence, Vinson explained, institutions could self-assess their status on the issue, chart a path toward improvement, and be rewarded for taking transformative action.

CLOSING STATEMENT

In closing the workshop, Fineberg observed that "there is a movement toward higher levels of rigor and transparency in science." He encouraged participants to continue to foster this movement and accelerate progress toward improving reproducibility and replicability across the biomedical research life cycle through transparent reporting.

Appendix A

References

Anderson, M. S., B. C. Martinson, and R. De Vries. 2007. Normative dissonance in science: Results from a national survey of U.S. scientists. *Journal of Empirical Research on Human Research Ethics* 2(4):3–14.

Bik, E. M., A. Casadevall, and F. C. Fang. 2016. The prevalence of inappropriate image duplication in biomedical research publications. *mBio* 7(3):e00809-16.

Bik, E. M., F. C. Fang, A. L. Kullas, R. J. Davis, and A. Casadevall. 2018. Analysis and correction of inappropriate image duplication: The *Molecular and Cellular Biology* experience. *Molecular and Cellular Biology* 38(20):e00309-18.

Bosk, C. L., M. Dixon-Woods, C. A. Goeschel, and P. J. Pronovost. 2009. Reality check for checklists. *Lancet* 374(9688):444–445.

Casadevall, A., and F. C. Fang. 2016. Rigorous science: A how-to guide. *mBio* 7(6):e01902-16.

Chan, A.-W., A. Hróbjartsson, M. T. Haahr, P. C. Gøtzsche, and D. G. Altman. 2004. Empirical evidence for selective reporting of outcomes in randomized trials: Comparison of protocols to published articles. *JAMA* 291:2457–2465.

Chan, A.-W., A. Hróbjartsson, K. J. Jørgensen, P. C. Gøtzsche, and D. G. Altman. 2008. Discrepancies in sample size calculations and data analyses reported in randomized trials: Comparison of publications with protocols. *BMJ* 337:a2299.

Chan, A.-W., J. M. Tetzlaff, D. G. Altman, K. Dickersin, and D. Moher. 2013a. SPIRIT 2013: New guidance for content of clinical trial protocols. *Lancet* 381(9861):91–92.

Chan, A.-W., J. M. Tetzlaff, D. G. Altman, A. Laupacis, P. C. Gøtzsche, K. Krleža-Jerić, A. Hróbjartsson, H. Mann, K. Dickersin, J. A. Berlin, C. J. Doré, W. R. Parulekar, W. S. Summerskill, T. Groves, K. F. Schulz, H. C. Sox, F. W. Rockhold, D. Rennie, and D. Moher. 2013b. SPIRIT 2013 statement: Defining standard protocol items for clinical trials. *Annals of Internal Medicine* 158(3):200–207.

Chan, A.-W., J. M. Tetzlaff, P. C. Gøtzsche, D. G. Altman, H. Mann, J. A. Berlin, K. Dickersin, A. Hróbjartsson, K. F. Schulz, W. R. Parulekar, K. Krleza-Jeric, A. Laupacis, and D. Moher. 2013c. SPIRIT 2013 explanation and elaboration: Guidance for protocols of clinical trials. *BMJ* 346:e7586.

Chan, A.-W., A. Pello, J. Kitchen, A. Axentiev, J. I. Virtanen, A. Liu, and E. Hemminki. 2017. Association of trial registration with reporting of primary outcomes in protocols and publications. *JAMA* 318(17):1709–1711.

Chuang, K. V., and M. J. Keiser. 2018. Adversarial controls for scientific machine learning. *ACS Chemical Biology* 13(10):2819–2821.

Collins, F. S., and L. A. Tabak. 2014. Policy: NIH plans to enhance reproducibility. *Nature* 505(7485):612–613.

Fanelli, D., J. P. A. Ioannidis, and S. Goodman. 2018. Improving the integrity of published science: An expanded taxonomy of retractions and corrections. *European Journal of Clinical Investigation* 48(4).

Gawande, A. 2009. *The checklist manifesto: How to get things right*. New York: Henry Holt and Company.

Getz, K., R. Zuckerman, A. Cropp, A. Hindle, R. Krauss, and K. Kaitin. 2011. Measuring the incidence, causes, and repercussions of protocol amendments. *Drug Information Journal* 45:265–275.

Hróbjartsson, A., J. Pildal, A.-W. Chan, M. T. Haahr, D. G. Altman, and P. C. Gøtzsche. 2009. Reporting on blinding in trial protocols and corresponding publications was often inadequate but rarely contradictory. *Journal of Clinical Epidemiology* 62:967–973.

Hudson, K. L., M. S. Lauer, and F. S. Collins. 2016. Toward a new era of trust and transparency in clinical trials. *JAMA* 316(13):1353–1354.

Ioannidis, J. P. 2005. Why most published research findings are false. *PLOS Medicine* 2(8):e124.

Jamieson, K. H., M. McNutt, V. Kiermer, and R. Sever. 2019. Signaling the trustworthiness of science. *Proceedings of the National Academy of Sciences in the United States of America* 116(39):19231–19236.

Kiley, R., T. Peatfield, J. Hansen, and R. Reddington. 2017. Data sharing from clinical trials—a research funder's perspective. *New England Journal of Medicine* 377:1990–1992.

Landis, S. C., S. G. Amara, K. Asadullah, C. P. Austin, R. Blumenstein, E. W. Bradley, R. G. Crystal, R. B. Darnell, R. J. Ferrante, H. Fillit, R. Finkelstein, M. Fisher, H. E. Gendelman, R. M. Golub, J. L. Goudreau, R. A. Gross, A. K. Gubitz, S. E. Hesterlee, D. W. Howells, J. Huguenard, K. Kelner, W. Koroshetz, D. Krainc, S. E. Lazic, M. S. Levine, M. R. Macleod, J. M. McCall, R. T. Moxley 3rd, K. Narasimhan, L. J. Noble, S. Perrin, J. D. Porter, O. Steward, E. Unger, U. Utz, and S. D. Silberberg. 2012. A call for transparent reporting to optimize the predictive value of preclinical research. *Nature* 490(7419):187–191.

Macleod, M. R., H. B. van der Worp, E. S. Sena, D. W. Howells, U. Dirnagl, and G. A. Donnan. 2008. Evidence for the efficacy of NXY-059 in experimental focal cerebral ischaemia is confounded by study quality. *Stroke* 39(10):2824–2829.

Mayo-Wilson, E., K. Vander Ley, K. Dickersin, and M. Helfand. 2017. *Patient-Centered Outcomes Research Institute (PCORI) Methodology Standards to improve the design and reporting of research*. Abstract for poster presentation at the Eighth International Congress on Peer Review and Scientific Publication, Chicago, IL. https://peerreviewcongress.org/prc17-0326 (accessed November 20, 2019).

McNutt, M., 2014. Journals unite for reproducibility. *Science* 346(6210):679.

Mhaskar, R., B. Djulbegovic, A. Magazin, H. P. Soares, and A. Kumar. 2012. Published methodological quality of randomized controlled trials does not reflect the actual quality assessed in protocols. *Journal of Clinical Epidemiology* 65:602–609.

NASEM (National Academies of Sciences, Engineering, and Medicine). 2017. *Fostering integrity in research*. Washington, DC: The National Academies Press.

NASEM. 2018. *Open science by design: Realizing a vision for 21st century research*. Washington, DC: The National Academies Press.

NASEM. 2019. *Reproducibility and replicability in science*. Washington, DC: The National Academies Press.

Nature Research. 2018. *Nature reproducibility survey 2017*. https://doi.org/10.6084/m9.figshare.6139937.v4.

Nosek, B. A., G. Alter, G. C. Banks, D. Borsboom, S. D. Bowman, S. J. Breckler, S. Buck, C. D. Chambers, G. Chin, G. Christensen, M. Contestabile, A. Dafoe, E. Eich, J. Freese, R. Glennerster, D. Goroff, D. P. Green, B. Hesse, M. Humphreys, J. Ishiyama, D. Karlan, A. Kraut, A. Lupia, P. Mabry, T. Madon, N. Malhotra, E. Mayo-Wilson, M. McNutt, E. Miguel, E. Levy Paluck, U. Simonsohn, C. Soderberg, B. A. Spellman, J. Turitto, G. VandenBos, S. Vazire, E. J. Wagenmakers, R. Wilson, and T. Yarkoni. 2015. Promoting an open research culture. *Science* 348(6242):1422–1425.

NPQIP (Nature Publishing Group Quality in Publishing) Collaborative Group. 2019. Did a change in *Nature* journals' editorial policy for life sciences research improve reporting? *BMJ Open Science* 3:e000035.

PCORI (Patient-Centered Outcomes Research Institute). 2019. *PCORI Methodology Standards*. https://www.pcori.org/methodology-standards (accessed November 20, 2019).

Pildal, J., A.-W. Chan, A. Hróbjartsson, E. Forfang, D. G. Altman, and P. C. Gøtzsche. 2005. Comparison of descriptions of allocation concealment in trial protocols and the published reports: Cohort study. *BMJ* 330:1049.

Platt, J. R. 1964. Strong inference: Certain systematic methods of scientific thinking may produce much more rapid progress than others. *Science* 146(3642):347–353.

Prinz, F., T. Schlange, and K. Asadullah. 2011. Believe it or not: How much can we rely on published data on potential drug targets? *Nature Review Drug Discovery* 10(9):712.

Russ, H., S. Busta, A. Riedel, G. Zöllner, and B. Jost. 2009. Evaluation of clinical trials by ethics committees in Germany: Experience of applicants with the review of requests for opinion of the ethics committees—results of a survey among members of the German Association of Research-Based Pharmaceutical Companies (VFA). *German Medical Science* 7:Doc07.

Scharf, O., and A. D. Colevas. 2006. Adverse event reporting in publications compared with sponsor database for cancer clinical trials. *Journal of Clinical Oncology* 24:3933–3938.

Sena, E. S., H. B. van der Worp, P. M. W. Bath, D. W. Howells, and M. R. Macleod. 2010. Publication bias in reports of animal stroke studies leads to major overstatement of efficacy. *PLOS Biology* 8(3):e1000344.

Silberberg, S. D., D. C. Crawford, R. Finkelstein, W. J. Koroshetz, R. D. Blank, H. H. Freeze, H. H. Garrison, and Y. R. Seger. 2017. Shake up conferences. *Nature* 548(7666):153–154.

Tang, Z., K. V. Chuang, C. DeCarli, L. W. Jin, L. Beckett, M. J. Keiser, and B. N. Dugger. 2019. Interpretable classification of Alzheimer's disease pathologies with a convolutional neural network pipeline. *Nature Communications* 10(1):2173.

Turner, L., L. Shamseer, D. G. Altman, L. Weeks, J. Peters, T. Kober, S. Dias, K. F. Schulz, A. C. Plint, and D. Moher. 2012. Consolidated standards of reporting trials (CONSORT) and the completeness of reporting of randomised controlled trials (RCTs) published in medical journals. *Cochrane Database of Systematic Reviews* 11:MR000030.

Williams, C. L., A. Casadevall, and S. Jackson. 2019. Figure errors, sloppy science, and fraud: Keeping eyes on your data. *Journal of Clinical Investigation* 129(5):1805–1807.

Appendix B

Background Discussion Document: Selected Guidelines for Transparent Reporting

SELECTED GUIDELINES FOR TRANSPARENT REPORTING

The purpose of this document is to help inform workshop discussions on improving the harmonization of guidelines for transparent reporting across journals and funding agencies so that biomedical researchers propose and report data in a consistent manner. This discussion document was compiled based on criteria described in the Transparency and Openness Promotion (TOP) guidelines;[1] the National Academies of Sciences, Engineering, and Medicine report on *Reproducibility and Replicability in Science;*[2] and the National Institutes of Health (NIH) policy on Enhancing Reproducibility through Rigor and Transparency.[3] Each of the guidelines summarized below has a different scope and purpose.

> *Rather than a comprehensive comparison of the several guidelines, this document indicates the criteria related to transparent reporting that are covered by the various guidelines. It is intended as a background for the workshop discussion.*

[1] Available at https://cos.io/top (accessed January 12, 2020).

[2] Available at https://www.nap.edu/catalog/25303/reproducibility-and-replicability-in-science (accessed January 12, 2020).

[3] Available at https://grants.nih.gov/policy/reproducibility/index.htm (accessed January 12, 2020).

BRIEF DESCRIPTIONS OF GUIDELINES SUMMARIZED

- The Animal Research: Reporting In Vivo Experiments (ARRIVE) guidelines recommend criteria for the reporting of primary research using animals. The guidelines were based on the Consolidated Standards of Reporting Trials (CONSORT) guidelines, but cover diverse study types. They were developed by the National Centre for the Replacement, Refinement and Reduction of Animals in Research (NC3Rs), and were first published in *PLOS Biology* in 2010. The ARRIVE guidelines are currently being revised; a preprint of the revised ARRIVE guidelines and the accompanying Explanation and Elaboration document are available on BioRxiv, respectively at https://www.biorxiv.org/content/10.1101/703181v1 and at https://www.biorxiv.org/content/10.1101/703355v1.
- The CONSORT statement recommends information to include when reporting a randomized trial; was developed by an international group of trialists, methodologists, and medical journal editors; and was first published in *JAMA* in 1996 and last revised in 2010 and published in multiple journals. For more information, see http://www.consort-statement.org.
- The **DRAFT** materials, design, analysis, and reporting (MDAR) checklist for authors represents a generic set of minimum requirements applicable to all reporting studies in the life sciences for the explicit purpose of increasing transparent reporting and reproducibility, developed by the MDAR working group specifically seeking common reporting points from across multiple journals. The checklist is being pilot tested by volunteer journals, and therefore has not been published at the time of this writing. The statement of task is available at https://osf.io/preprints/metaarxiv/9sm4x.
- NIH policies:
  - "Data Sharing" policy, developed by NIH, to encourage data generated with NIH funding to be "made as widely and freely available as possible while safeguarding the privacy of participants, and protecting confidential and proprietary data." The policy requires a data sharing plan for final research data generated on grants of $500,000 or more, and was implemented in 2003. For more information, see https://grants.nih.gov/grants/policy/data_sharing.
  - "Dissemination of NIH-Funded Clinical Trial Information" policy, developed by NIH and implemented in 2017, mandates that all clinical trials funded in part or in whole by NIH must be registered at ClinicalTrials.gov. The policy also requires that summary results be posted to ClinicalTrials.gov. For more infor-

  mation, see https://grants.nih.gov/grants/guide/notice-files/not-od-16-149.html.
  - "Enhancing Reproducibility through Rigor and Transparency" policy, developed by NIH, to clarify expectations for grantees and reviewers in describing or assessing proposed studies in applications and progress reports, announced in 2015 and implemented in 2016. For more information, see https://grants.nih.gov/policy/reproducibility/index.htm.
- The Preferred Reporting Items for Systematic Reviews and Meta-Analyses (PRISMA) statement recommends an evidence-based minimum set of reporting elements for systematic reviews and meta-analyses; was developed by an international group; and was first published in 2009 in multiple journals (*PLOS Medicine, Annals of Internal Medicine, BMJ, Journal of Clinical Epidemiology*, and *Open Medicine*). For more information, see http://www.prisma-statement.org.
- The Standard Protocol Items: Recommendations for Interventional Trials (SPIRIT) statement, developed by an international collaboration of trialists, methodologists, journal editors, and ethicists, recommends minimum content to include in clinical trial protocols, from study enrollment through closeout, first published in the *Annals of Internal Medicine* and *BMJ* in 2013. For more information, see https://www.spirit-statement.org.
- The TOP guidelines describe eight modular standards of transparency that journals can select from to introduce policy and best practices at their publication; was developed by the Center for Open Science with input from journals, funders, and professional societies; and was first published in *Science* in 2015. See https://cos.io/top for information about TOP, including a summary table and links to complete policy language.

Legend
Criterion covered: Dark boxes
Criterion partially covered: Gray boxes
Criterion not covered: White boxes

	ARRIVE *Primary Research in Animals*	CONSORT *Randomized Trials*
STUDY CHARACTERISTICS		
Code availability[2]	Not covered	Not covered
Data availability[2,3]	Covered	Covered
Data citation[2,3]	Covered	Not covered
STUDY METHODS		
Analytical methods: attrition, statistical precision, statistical power[2,3]	Covered	Covered
Plan for analytical decisions/preregistration[2,3]	Covered	Covered
Animal use/sex as a biologic variable[4]	Covered	Not covered
Details of in-laboratory study replication[3]	Covered	Not covered
Details of study methods, computation, and associated parameters[2,3]	Covered	Covered
Ethics[2,5]	Covered	Not covered
Information on computational environment (e.g., operating system, library dependencies)[3]	Not covered	Not covered
Materials availability discussed[2,3]	Covered	Not covered
Material authentication required[4]	Not covered	Not covered
Methods and protocols[2,3,4]	Covered	Covered
Sample definition[2]	Covered	Covered
RESULTS AND DISCUSSION		
Adherence to community standards[2]	Not covered	Not covered
Discussion of uncertainty[3]	Covered	Covered
Discussion on generality constraints[3]	Covered	Covered
Discuss/assess rigor of prior research[4]	Not covered	Not covered
Dual use research of concern*	Not covered	Covered

1. NIH policies represented include Data Sharing Policy, Dissemination of NIH-Funded Clinical Trial Information, and Rigor and Transparency.
2. Based on criteria described in the Transparency and Openness Promotion (TOP) guidelines, https://cos.io/top.
3. Based on criteria described in the National Academies report *Reproducibility and Replicability in Science.*

DRAFT MDAR *Compilation of Multiple Life Science Journals*	NIH Policies[1] *Preclinical and Clinical Research*	PRISMA *Meta-analyses*	SPIRIT *Clinical Trial Protocols*	TOP Guidelines *Modular Publishing Standards*
[redacted]			[redacted]	[redacted]
[redacted]		[redacted]	[redacted]	[redacted]
[redacted]		[redacted]		[redacted]
[redacted]	[redacted]	[redacted]	[redacted]	[redacted]
[redacted]	[redacted]			
[redacted]				[redacted]
[redacted]	[redacted]	[redacted]	[redacted]	[redacted]
[redacted]	[redacted]		[redacted]	[redacted]
[redacted]			[redacted]	[redacted]
[redacted]	[redacted]			
[redacted]	[redacted]	[redacted]	[redacted]	[redacted]
[redacted]	[redacted]		[redacted]	[redacted]
[redacted]				[redacted]
		[redacted]		
	[redacted]	[redacted]		
[redacted]	[redacted]	[redacted]	[redacted]	

4. Based on criteria described in the NIH policy on Enhancing Reproducibility through Rigor and Transparency.
5. Covered by multiple NIH policies and offices, including Human Subjects Research policies and the NIH Office of Laboratory Animal Welfare.
* Covered by U.S. government Policy for Institutional Oversight of Life Sciences Dual Use Research of Concern.

Appendix C

Workshop Agenda

Enhancing Scientific Reproducibility in Biomedical Research Through Transparent Reporting—A Workshop

September 25–26, 2019

National Academy of Sciences Building, Lecture Room
2101 Constitution Avenue, NW, Washington, DC 20418

An ad hoc committee of the National Academies of Sciences, Engineering, and Medicine is convening a public workshop to discuss the current state of transparency in reporting preclinical biomedical research (e.g., disclosure of the availability and location of data, materials, analysis, and methodology) and to explore the possibility of improving the harmonization of guidelines across journals and funding agencies so that biomedical researchers propose and report data in a consistent manner. This workshop is sponsored by the Cell Press, *The Lancet*, the National Institutes of Health, and Nature Research.

WORKSHOP OBJECTIVES:

- Highlight current efforts by researchers, institutions, funders, and journals to increase transparency in proposing and reporting preclinical biomedical research;
- Consider lessons learned from field-specific best practices for increased transparency in reporting rigor elements (i.e., research design, methodology, analysis, interpretation, and reporting of results) that are generalizable across biomedical research domains;
- Discuss journal and funder assessments of researchers' adherence to transparent reporting guidelines, including a discussion of the effectiveness of checklists;
- Discuss opportunities for improving the consistency of reporting guidelines and requirements for rigor and transparency by journals, funders, and institutions across the biomedical research life cycle; and
- Consider approaches to compare reporting of rigor elements proposed in grant applications with those included in publications.

DAY 1: September 25, 2019

8:00 a.m.	Breakfast available outside the Lecture Room
8:30 a.m.	**Welcome and opening remarks** HARVEY FINEBERG, *Workshop Chair* President Gordon and Betty Moore Foundation **Highlights and related recommendations from the National Academies report on *Reproducibility and Replicability in Science***
9:15 a.m.	**Q&A with audience**

SESSION I — CULTIVATING TRANSPARENT REPORTING IN BIOMEDICAL RESEARCH

Session Objectives:

- Highlight current efforts by researchers, institutions, funders, and journals to increase transparency in proposing and reporting preclinical biomedical research.

- Discuss the incentives, disincentives, challenges, and opportunities for researchers when it comes to transparent reporting of preclinical biomedical research (e.g., pressure to publish, institutional resources, training, funding).
- Discuss experience with implementation of policies to encourage transparent reporting across the biomedical research life cycle.
- Consider the role of stakeholders in supporting a cultural shift toward transparent reporting in preclinical biomedical research. *For more information on cultural barriers as sources of non-reproducibility, see p. 58, p. 97, and p. 104 of the National Academies'* Reproducibility and Replicability in Science *consensus study report.*

9:30 a.m. **Opening remarks by session moderator**
ALEXA MCCRAY
Professor of Medicine
Harvard Medical School

9:40 a.m. **A researcher (early career) perspective**
YARIMAR CARRASQUILLO
Investigator
National Center for Complementary and Integrative Health, National Institutes of Health (NIH)

9:55 a.m. **A researcher/researcher support perspective**
BRIAN NOSEK
Co-founder
Center for Open Science

10:10 a.m. **A researcher (later career)/society publisher perspective**
ARTURO CASADEVALL
Professor, Molecular Microbiology and Immunology, Johns Hopkins University
Editor-in-Chief, *mBio*

10:25 a.m. **An NIH perspective**
CARRIE WOLINETZ
Acting Chief of Staff and Associate Director for Science Policy
Office of the Director, NIH

10:40 a.m. **Audience Q&A with the panel**

Discussion questions:

- What forces are influencing the culture of biomedical research, and how is it changing?
- What actions could influence practice and support a cultural shift toward more transparent reporting?
- What influence might transparent reporting or required reporting of rigor elements have on grant applications? Is there a role for preregistration of preclinical studies?

11:10 a.m. **BREAK**

SESSION II ANSWERING THE CALL FOR CHANGE: LESSONS LEARNED AND BEST PRACTICES

Session Objectives:

- Consider lessons learned from institutional and/or field-specific best practices for increased transparency in reporting rigor elements (i.e., research design, methodology, analysis, interpretation, and reporting of results) that are generalizable across biomedical research domains.
- Consider available tools and best practices for increased transparent reporting that support researchers and are generalizable across biomedical research domains.
- Discuss the roles of educational institutions, professional societies, researchers, and funders in improving computational reproducibility (*Reproducibility and Replicability in Science* Recommendation 6-6).
- Discuss how funding agencies and organizations could invest in research and development of open source, usable tools, and infrastructure that support reproducibility for a broad range of studies across different domains in a seamless fashion, as well as in outreach to inform and train researchers on best practices (*Reproducibility and Replicability in Science* Recommendation 6-1).

11:30 a.m. **Opening remarks by session moderator**
VERONIQUE KIERMER
Executive Editor
Public Library of Science (PLOS)

11:40 a.m.	**A clinical researcher perspective: Lessons from the SPIRIT initiative** AN-WEN CHAN Phelan Scientist, Women's College Research Institute Associate Professor, University of Toronto
11:50 a.m.	**An institution perspective** GEETA SWAMY Vice Dean for Scientific Integrity Associate Vice President for Research Duke University
12:00 p.m.	**A funder perspective** MAGALI HAAS Chief Executive Officer and President Cohen Veterans Bioscience
12:10 p.m.	**Moderated panel discussion among speakers**
12:30 p.m.	**Audience Q&A with the panel**

Discussion questions:

- How can challenges with preregistration, image analysis, cell line authentication, statistical analysis, or other rigor elements be addressed?
- What actions can institutions or professional societies take to educate and support their constituents on best practices? How could this information be best provided?
- How might funding agencies and organizations invest in development of open source reusable tools and infrastructure to support transparent reporting seamlessly across different domains?
- What actions could funding agencies and organizations take to inform, train, and support researchers on best practices in transparent reporting?
- What has been learned from open access mandates and from implementing policies around sharing data in preclinical research? How could those lessons inform transparent reporting guidance and adoption?

1:00 p.m.	**BREAK** (Lunch available outside the Lecture Room)

SESSION III STAKEHOLDER PERSPECTIVES ON CHECKLISTS AND GUIDELINES

Session Objectives:

- Discuss journal and funder assessments of researchers' adherence to transparent reporting guidelines, including discussion of the effectiveness of checklists.
    - Highlight empirical assessments of checklist application from funders, journals, and researchers; and
    - Consider practical application and effectiveness of checklists and guidelines to encourage or require transparent reporting of preclinical biomedical research.
- Discuss how funders could require thoughtful discussion in grant applications of how uncertainties will be evaluated, along with any relevant issues regarding replicability and computational reproducibility (*Reproducibility and Replicability in Science* Recommendation 6-9).
- Discuss how journals and scientific societies could disclose their policies relevant to achieving reproducibility and replicability, and how journals could be encouraged to set and implement desired standards of reproducibility and replicability and adopt policies to reduce the likelihood of non-replicability (*Reproducibility and Replicability in Science* Recommendation 6-7).

2:00 p.m. **Opening remarks by session moderator**
BARRY COLLER
Physician-in-Chief, Vice President for Medical Affairs, and David Rockefeller Professor
The Rockefeller University

2:10 p.m. **The checklist approach at life science journals—challenges and opportunities**
SOWMYA SWAMINATHAN
Head of Editorial Policy
Nature Research

MALCOLM MACLEOD
Professor
University of Edinburgh

2:30 p.m. **An NIH funder perspective**
SHAI SILBERBERG
Director, Research Quality
National Institute of Neurological Disorders and Stroke, NIH

2:40 p.m. **Moderated panel discussion among speakers**

3:10 p.m. **Audience Q&A with the panel**

Discussion questions:

- How valuable are checklists? How valuable is guidance such as the CONSORT statement? What are observed challenges to adherence, and how could they be addressed?
- How could checklists be improved and/or complemented to further encourage transparent reporting?
- What resources do researchers need to be able to submit proposals, publish, or otherwise report on specific rigor elements?
- How might funders require thoughtful discussion in grant applications of how uncertainties (e.g., in measurement, computation, knowledge, modeling, or methods of analysis) will be evaluated by researchers?
- Should scientific societies be encouraged to develop policies relevant to transparent reporting?

SESSION IV PART 1 — TOWARD MINIMAL REPORTING STANDARDS FOR PRECLINICAL BIOMEDICAL RESEARCH

Session Objective:

- Discuss opportunities for improving the consistency of reporting guidelines and requirements for rigor and transparency by journals, funders, and institutions across the biomedical research life cycle.

4:00 p.m. **Discussion with audience on potential steps stakeholders could take to support harmonizing reporting guidelines**

HARVEY FINEBERG, *Workshop Chair and session moderator*
President
Gordon and Betty Moore Foundation

BENEDICT KOLBER
Associate Professor
Duquesne University

RICHARD NAKAMURA
Former Director (Retired)
Center for Scientific Review, NIH

FRANKLIN SAYRE
STEM Librarian
Thompson Rivers University

VALDA VINSON
Editor, Research
Science

5:00 p.m. **ADJOURN WORKSHOP DAY 1**

DAY 2: September 26, 2019

8:00 a.m. Breakfast available outside the Lecture Room

8:30 a.m. **Welcome and overview of day 1**
HARVEY FINEBERG, *Workshop Chair*
President
Gordon and Betty Moore Foundation

9:00 a.m. **Keynote address**
MARCIA MCNUTT
President
National Academy of Sciences

9:20 a.m. **Q&A session**

9:30 a.m.	**BREAK**

SESSION IV PART 2	TOWARD MINIMAL REPORTING STANDARDS FOR PRECLINICAL BIOMEDICAL RESEARCH

Session Objectives:

- Consider approaches to compare reporting of rigor elements proposed in grant applications to those included in publications.
- Suggest stakeholder actions to encourage transparent reporting and practical next steps toward establishing minimal reporting standards for preclinical biomedical research.

10:00 a.m. **Opening remarks by session moderator**
HARVEY FINEBERG, *Workshop Chair*
President
Gordon and Betty Moore Foundation

10:10 a.m. **An early career researcher perspective**
MICHAEL KEISER
Assistant Professor
University of California, San Francisco

10:20 a.m. **An institution perspective**
MELISSA RETHLEFSEN
Associate Dean, George A. Smathers Libraries
Fackler Director, Health Science Center Libraries
University of Florida

10:30 a.m. **A research educator perspective**
STEVEN GOODMAN
Professor of Medicine and Health Research and Policy
Co-director, Meta-Research Innovation Center at Stanford
Stanford University

10:40 a.m. **Moderated panel discussion among speakers**

11:10 a.m. **Small group table discussion and reporting**

Discussion questions:

- What actions should funders, researchers, institutions, and journals take to drive widespread adoption of minimal reporting standards?

- Are reporting categories in guidelines for publishing (e.g., materials, design, analysis, and reporting) relevant for funders? For institutions? For small publishers/professional societies?
- What other information or reporting categories would be relevant?
- How should funders instruct reviewers of grant applications to reinforce transparent reporting? How much information should funders request, that is, to what level of detail, in grant applications? Is it possible to obtain sufficient information about transparent reporting in grant applications without dramatic expansion of the application?

12:25 p.m. **Workshop wrap-up and concluding discussion with audience**

12:30 p.m. **ADJOURN WORKSHOP DAY 2**